A DENTAL PRACTITIONER HANDBOOK
SERIES EDITED BY DONALD D. DERRICK, D.D.S., L.D.S. R.C.S.

FRACTURES OF THE MIDDLE THIRD OF THE FACIAL SKELETON

H. C. KILLEY
F.D.S. R.C.S.(Eng.), F.D.S., H.D.D. R.C.S.(Edin.),
L.R.C.P.(Lond.), M.R.C.S.(Eng.), F.I.C.S.

Professor of Oral Surgery, London University.
Head of Department of Oral Surgery,
Institute of Dental Surgery.
Hon. Consultant in Oral Surgery, Eastman Dental Hospital
and Westminster Hospital Teaching Group.
Formerly: Consultant in Oral Surgery and Maxillo-facial Injuries,
Plastic and Jaw Unit, Rooksdown House, Basingstoke,
Holy Cross Hospital, Haslemere,
Aldershot General Hospital,
and Queen Mary's Hospital, Roehampton

THIRD EDITION

BRISTOL: JOHN WRIGHT & SONS LTD.
1977

First edition, 1965
Second edition, 1971
Revised reprint, 1974
Third edition, 1977

ISBN 0 7236 0459 2

PRINTED IN GREAT BRITAIN BY HENRY LING LTD., A SUBSIDIARY OF JOHN WRIGHT & SONS LTD., AT THE DORSET PRESS, DORCHESTER

PREFACE TO THE THIRD EDITION

SINCE the Second Edition of this monograph was published in 1971 there have been no important advances in the interpretation of the surgical anatomy and in the diagnosis of fractures of the middle third of the facial skeleton, and the general principles of treatment are also unaltered. Only minimal revision of the main body of the text has therefore been necessary. However, there is increasing interest in the isolated orbital floor fracture and the section that deals with this type of injury has been expanded. Important new references on the subject have been added to the Bibliography.

The multi-discipline approach to the treatment of patients with severe multiple injuries has recently become more firmly established. This policy has become necessary owing to the increasing severity and complexity of the injuries received as a result of road traffic accidents. This trend in treatment is leading to the gradual obsolescence of the traditional maxillo-facial or plastic and jaw units. These units were ideally staffed and equipped to deal with hard and soft tissue injuries of the face, but less capable of handling severe chest and abdominal injuries often associated with multiple fractures of the limbs. Accident centres have therefore been established at large hospitals and they are directed by specially trained accident surgeons with a background of general and orthopaedic surgery who call upon the skilled assistance of other specialists depending upon the nature of the surgical problem. In such centres specialist anaesthetists deal with the immediate resuscitation of the patient and supervise the intensive care. Medical specialists backed by biochemists advise upon the blood and fluid replacement problems. Many of the casualties have an associated head or eye injury and the neurosurgeon and ophthalmic surgeon undertake the care of such injuries. Plastic surgeons are called upon to treat severe facial lacerations and the maxillo-facial specialist is included in the team when there are facial fractures.

In a small book it is impossible to discuss in adequate detail the various important aspects of the multi-discipline approach to the treatment of casualties such as resuscitation and intensive care. The text is therefore devoted exclusively to the problems associated with the surgical anatomy, diagnosis and principles of treatment of fractures of the middle third of the facial skeleton.

It is hoped that the present volume will continue to be a useful introduction to the subject and that it contains an adequate amount of material for the higher examinations in dentistry.

1976   H. C. K.

PREFACE TO THE FIRST EDITION

ONE of the most serious injuries which the dental surgeon is called upon to diagnose and treat is a severe fracture of the middle third of the facial skeleton.

These cases are by no means uncommon and are caused principally by traffic accidents, motor-cyclists and motorists being more or less equally involved. At the present time these fractures appear to be increasing, probably due to the increase in road traffic and the fact that the introduction of safety devices, such as the crash helmet and the safety belt, preserve the life of many motor-cyclists and motorists who would otherwise have been killed at the time of the accident. This has resulted in more patients with extensive multiple injuries reaching hospital alive.

The specialist dental surgeon working in a hospital must, of necessity, be prepared to deal with such injuries, but any dental surgeon, especially if he is a motorist or works in the vicinity of one of the large arterial roads, may suddenly be confronted with an unconscious patient who has sustained a severe fracture of the middle third of the facial skeleton.

Life-saving measures to maintain the airway and control haemorrhage must be carried out immediately, and to perform this duty efficiently, the dental surgeon requires a clear understanding of the surgical anatomy of the part, together with the ability to observe and interpret the physical signs and so diagnose the exact nature of the injury.

H. C. K.

CONTENTS

CHAPTER   PAGE

I.—INTRODUCTION   9

II.—SURGICAL ANATOMY   11

III.—CLASSIFICATION   16

IV.—THE MANAGEMENT OF FRACTURES OF THE MIDDLE THIRD
OF THE FACIAL SKELETON   20

V.—HISTORY AND LOCAL EXAMINATION   25

VI.—CLINICAL FINDINGS IN THE VARIOUS TYPES OF FRACTURE   27
     Dento-alveolar Fractures   27
     Fractures of the Zygomatic Complex   28
     Isolated Orbital Floor Fractures   36
     Fractures of the Nasal Complex   38
     Le Fort I, Low-level, or Guérin Type Fractures   ..   40
     Le Fort II or Pyramidal Type Fractures   41
     Le Fort III, High-level, or Supra-zygomatic Fractures   44

VII.—CEREBROSPINAL FLUID RHINORRHOEA   48

VIII.—RADIOLOGY FOR FRACTURES OF THE MIDDLE THIRD OF THE
FACIAL SKELETON   50

IX.—OUTLINE OF DEFINITIVE TREATMENT OF FRACTURES OF THE
MIDDLE THIRD OF THE FACIAL SKELETON   51
     Dento-alveolar Fractures   51
     Zygomatic Complex Fractures   53
     Nasal Complex Fractures   58
     Le Fort I, II, and III Type Fractures   60
     Immobilization of Le Fort I, II, and III Type Fractures   62
     Outline of Definitive Procedures in Facial Fractures
         where Treatment has been delayed   72
     Post-operative Management of Fractures of the Middle
         Third of the Facial Skeleton   73
     Late Complications of Fractures of the Middle Third
         of the Facial Skeleton   74

     BIBLIOGRAPHY   77

     INDEX   85

ACKNOWLEDGEMENTS

My thanks are due to Mr. Lester Kay, M.D.S., F.D.S. R.C.S., L.R.C.P., M.R.C.S., Reader in Oral Surgery, Eastman Dental Hospital, for reading the script and for much helpful advice. My thanks are also due to Miss Archer, Medical Artist, Guy's Hospital, for *Figs.* 21, 22, 35, 36, 37, and 38, and to Mr. E. Pullen-Warner for *Figs.* 2, 3, and 8 and for *Fig.* 25. *Fig.* 31 was originally published in ' Maxillo-Facial Injuries ', H. C. Killey, *Hospital Medicine*, **2,** 917–928 (1968), and my thanks are due to the Editor for permission to reproduce it. *Fig.* 12 is published by kind permission of the Editor of the *Journal of the South African Dental Association*, where it was originally published in a paper entitled 'Fractures of the Zygomatic Arch', H. C. Killey and L. W. Kay, **23,** 391–394.

I am grateful to Mr. N. M. Potter and Mr. J. Morgan of the Eastman Dental Hospital, and to Mr. E. Ferrill of Queen Mary's Hospital, Roehampton, for the photography. Finally, my sincere thanks are due to my secretary Miss B. Richardson for her help in typing and arranging the script and to Mrs. B. Rayiru for secretarial assistance in the preparation of the revised reprint edition. Mrs. Clark kindly prepared the script for the Third Edition and I am most grateful to her.

FRACTURES OF THE MIDDLE THIRD OF THE FACIAL SKELETON

Chapter I

INTRODUCTION

THE facial skeleton can be roughly divided into three areas: the lower third or mandible, the upper third, which is formed by the frontal bone, and the middle third, an area extending downwards from the frontal bone to the level of the upper teeth or, if the patient is edentulous, the upper alveolus.

Fractures of the middle third area have also been called 'upper jaw fractures' or 'fractures of the maxilla', but in view of the fact that bones adjacent to the upper jaw are almost invariably involved in such injuries, these terms are not strictly accurate. Fractures of the middle third of the facial skeleton and/or the mandible are known as 'maxillo-facial injuries' and they are associated with varying degrees of involvement of the overlying soft tissues and such neighbouring structures as the eyes, nasal airways, paranasal sinuses, and tongue. They can vary in severity from a simple crack in the upper alveolus to a major disruption of the entire facial skeleton. The bones of the middle third of the facial skeleton present a superficial appearance of strength but they are, in fact, comparatively fragile and they fragment and comminute easily. In view of the fact that they articulate and interdigitate in a most complex fashion, it is difficult to fracture one bone without disrupting its neighbours. This gross comminution is difficult to visualize, for middle third injuries are usually closed fractures, but in a severe Le Fort III type fracture the middle third area may be comminuted into 60 or 70 separate fragments.

INCIDENCE

Maxillo-facial injuries are not particularly common, but it is difficult to arrive at any accurate estimate of their incidence, for many of the authorities who have reviewed series of such injuries do not state the period over which the cases were collected. Mallett (1950) reviewed 2124 cases of jaw fracture treated at the Boston City Hall Hospital from 1919 to 1948. Harnisch (1960) collected 532 fractures between 1952 and 1957 at the Rudolf Virchow Hospital in Berlin. Lindstrom (1960), of the Department of Dentistry of the University of Finland, reviewed 649 patients seen from 1948 to 1958. One of the largest series is that of Schuchardt and others (1966) of Hamburg, Germany, for in the period 1946–1957 they collected 1566 facial fractures and from 1958 to 1963 they reviewed a further 1335 cases, a total of 2901 facial fractures. In this series 774 fractures involved the middle third and 156 the middle third and mandible, a total of 930 cases. Rowe and Killey (1968) analysed 1500 facial fractures, and in this series 501 involved the middle third and 128 affected both the mandible and the middle third, a total of 629 fractures of the middle third. However, Kelly and Harrigan (1975) analysed 3324 patients admitted with fractures of the facial skeleton, and of 4317 fractures only 594 involved the middle third of the facial skeleton.

Aetiology

Any severe trauma can cause a fracture of the middle third of the facial skeleton, but the majority of these injuries are caused by road traffic accidents. In a series of 629 middle third injuries (Rowe and Killey, 1968), 296 or 47·05 per cent resulted from accidents to two- or four-wheel vehicles.

CHAPTER II

SURGICAL ANATOMY

THE middle third of the facial skeleton is defined as an area bounded superiorly by a line drawn across the skull from the zygomatico-frontal suture across the fronto-nasal and fronto-maxillary sutures to the zygomatico-frontal suture on the opposite side, and inferiorly by the occlusal plane of the upper teeth, or, if the patient is edentulous, by the upper alveolar ridge. It extends backwards as far as the frontal bone above and the body of the sphenoid below, and the pterygoid plates of the sphenoid are usually involved in any severe fracture.

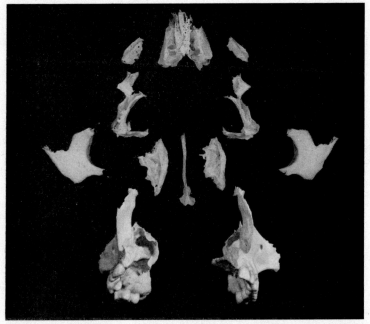

Fig. 1.—The bones of the middle third of the facial skeleton. Note that they are all comparatively fragile and that they must obviously articulate in a most complex fashion. From above down they are the ethmoid and its attached conchae, flanked by the two lacrimal bones. Next, the palatine bones and beneath them, from without in, the zygomatic bones, the inferior nasal conchae, and the vomer. The two maxillae are photographed to demonstrate the maxillary sinuses.

The middle third of the facial skeleton is made up of the following bones:—

1.   Two maxillae;
2.   Two zygomatic bones;

3. Two zygomatic processes of the temporal bones;
4. Two palatine bones;
5. Two nasal bones;
6. Two lacrimal bones;
7. The vomer;
8. The ethmoid and its attached conchae;
9. Two inferior conchae;
10. The pterygoid plates of the sphenoid.

The frontal bone, the body and greater and lesser wings of the sphenoid are not usually fractured. In fact, they are protected to a considerable extent by the cushioning effect achieved as the fracturing force crushes the comparatively weak bones comprising the middle third of the facial skeleton.

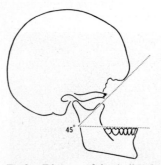

Fig. 2.—Diagram of the skull and mandible with the middle third of the facial skeleton removed. It will be seen that the frontal bone and body of the sphenoid bone form an inclined plane which lies at an angle of about 45° to the occlusal plane. In the Le Fort II and III types of fracture the bones of the middle third of the facial skeleton are driven down this inclined plane and the oral airway is occluded when the tissues of the soft palate meet the tongue.

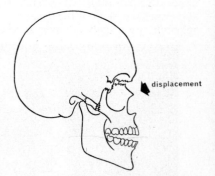

Fig. 3.—Downwards and backwards displacement of the bones of the middle third of the facial skeleton down the inclined plane formed by the frontal bone and body of the sphenoid (see Fig. 2) resulting in occlusion of the oral airway. The downwards displacement of the upper jaw pushes the mandible to the open position.

The surgical anatomy of the area is very complicated because it is intimately associated with a number of important structures such as the brain, the cranial nerves, the orbits, the paranasal sinuses, the nares, and the mouth. The most important features of the surgical anatomy of the middle third of the facial skeleton are as follows:—

1. The middle third of the facial skeleton is made up of a considerable number of bones, and it is difficult, if not impossible, to fracture one of these bones without involving the other bones to which it is attached.

2. Although the facial bones appear to be strong, they are, in fact, fragile. (*Fig.* 1.)

The middle third of the facial skeleton is designed to withstand the force of mastication from below and all the bony lines of strength are arranged to carry force from the upper teeth and distribute it over the base of the skull. This can be demonstrated if the comparatively thin areas of bone comprising the outer walls of the maxillary sinuses are removed from the maxillae, when it will be seen that the middle third of the facial skeleton consists of a series of bony struts passing upwards from the upper teeth to the base of the skull. Although these bony struts can withstand considerable force from below, they are easily fractured by relatively trivial forces applied laterally, such as a blow on the bridge of the nose or across the face above the apices of the upper teeth.

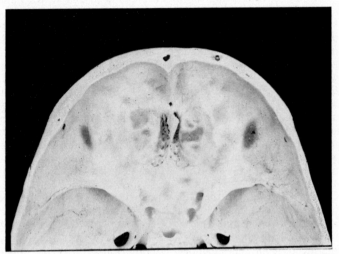

Fig. 4.—View of the cribriform plate of the ethmoid. This fragile bone is fractured in Le Fort II and III type fractures and also in severe injuries of the naso-ethmoidal complex.

It is, therefore, not surprising that facial fractures may occur as the result of slight trauma, and it is not uncommon to find a patient with an extensive fracture following a blow across the bridge of the nose which was not sufficiently severe to cause loss of consciousness.

3. If the bones comprising the middle third of the facial skeleton are removed from a skull, it will be seen that the frontal bone and body of the sphenoid form an inclined plane which slopes downwards and backwards from the frontal bone at an angle of about 45° to the occlusal plane of the upper teeth.

The bones of the middle third of the facial skeleton articulate with these strong foundation bones and when force is applied to them, they are crushed or sheared off the cranial base and are forced down the inclined plane formed by the frontal and sphenoid bones (*Fig. 2*). The bones of the middle third of the facial skeleton absorb most of the fracturing force and so protect the underlying bones of the skull from all but overwhelming trauma. As the facial bones are driven down the inclined plane, the face is pushed in and the posterior teeth of the maxillae push open the mandible (*Fig. 3*). This leads to great lengthening of the face. Many of these patients on admission complain of trismus but, in point of fact, the mouth is already open widely and closure of the lower jaw can only be effected by elevating the upper jaw.

As the upper jaw is displaced downwards and backwards, the soft palate is pushed down upon the dorsum of the tongue. This prevents the patient from breathing through the mouth and, as the nares are blocked already by blood-clot, the patient will rapidly suffocate unless urgent measures are taken to restore an airway. As a first-aid measure, two fingers can be hooked around the back of the hard palate, and the upper jaw pulled upwards and forwards along the inclined plane to enable the patient to breathe through the mouth.

4. Fractures of the middle third of the facial skeleton are invariably multiple, and in a Le Fort III type fracture there may be as many as sixty or seventy fragments. It is sometimes difficult to visualize this fact as the soft tissues of the face are usually not lacerated and the fractures are not compound.

5. Damage to the infra-orbital nerve may occur with zygomatic, Le Fort II, and Le Fort III fractures either unilaterally or bilaterally and, depending upon whether there is a neurapraxia or a neurotmesis, recovery may take eight to eighteen months. Other nerves which may be damaged are the anterior, middle, and posterior superior dental nerves. Patients seldom notice anaesthesia of the gum at the time of injury, but if the distribution of these nerves is tested at a later date areas of anaesthesia will be found.

6. Comminution of the ethmoid occurs with Le Fort II and III fractures and some severe fractures of the nasal complex. This may lead to a dural tear and cerebrospinal fluid rhinorrhoea. (*Fig.* 4.) More rarely a profuse cerebrospinal rhinorrhoea occurs as a result of a fracture which passes through the base of the sphenoid, communicating with the sphenoidal sinus and through a crack in the roof of this structure with the cisterna chiasmatica.

7. Fractures involving the orbit may give rise to alteration in position of the globe of the eye. If the orbital floor is comminuted, there is a herniation of the periorbital fat into the maxillary sinus which may lead to an enophthalmos. Fractures of the orbital floor may result in the inferior oblique and the inferior rectus muscles being involved in the defect, or they can be bound down by subsequent fibrous tissue formation. This results in mechanical interference which prevents upward and outward rotation of the eye and causes vertical diplopia.

Alteration in the level of the globe of the eye will occur if the fracture passes above the origin or insertion of Lockwood's suspensory ligament. This fascial sling which cradles the globe of the eye passes from the lacrimal bone to be inserted into Whitnall's tubercle situated on the inner aspect of the zygomatic bone just below the zygomatico-frontal suture. If the fracture passes beneath Whitnall's tubercle there can be a severe drop in the zygomatic bone without any corresponding descent in the level of the eye. As the globe of the eye drops, the upper lid follows it downwards, giving rise to the physical sign known as 'hooding of the eye'. Alteration in the ocular level does not cause diplopia unless there is associated damage to any of the extra-ocular muscles or the nerves innervating those muscles.

8. As the middle third of the facial skeleton is pushed down the inclined plane formed by the frontal bone and the body of the sphenoid, the mandible is forced open with bilateral gagging of the molar teeth, retro-position of the upper incisors, and the occurrence of an anterior open bite.

9. If there is a depressed fracture of the zygomatic bones, they may impinge on the coronoid process on one or both sides and prevent lateral excursion of the mandible towards the fractured side. If the mouth was wide open at the time of injury, the zygomatic bone may be in such a position that the coronoid process impinges upon it and prevents mandibular closure.

10. If the naso-ethmoidal complex is shattered the nares are, of course, blocked with blood-clot.

11. In zygomatic complex and Le Fort II and III fractures, the maxillary sinuses are involved. Gross comminution of the antral walls occurs and on X-ray examination one or both antra appear opaque. A few days after the injury a fluid level may sometimes be seen. Apart from the routine reduction and repositioning of the fracture, no special treatment is required in the treatment of the antral wall fractures and about six weeks later X-rays will show apparently clear sinuses. Post-operative reviews of fractures of the middle third of the facial skeleton show no greater incidence of chronic antral infection in these cases than in the remainder of the population. Kreirler and Koch (1975) carried out an endoscopic study of the maxillary sinus after middle face fractures in 25 patients and found 35 per cent had chronic mucosal changes, but all were free of symptoms.

12. Le Fort II and III fractures and severe nasal complex injuries may involve the nasolacrimal duct, with resulting epiphora. This complication is not noticed at the time of injury, but may become apparent later.

13. The maxillae may be separated along their median palatal suture line by a cleaving blow directed up the centre of the upper jaw, or by a blow transmitted upwards via the mandibular teeth in patients having markedly overclosed bites.

14. The optic foramen is a ring of compact bone and in high-level or Le Fort III injuries fractures invariably occur around it, so that it is unusual for the optic nerve to be damaged directly as the result of a middle-third fracture. C. R. Stockdale (1959) has reported one case of fractured middle third complicated by loss of vision.

15. The degree and direction of the displacement of fragments in fractures of the middle third of the facial skeleton are brought about by the fracturing force. The muscles of facial expression which have their origin in the middle third of the facial skeleton are inserted into skin and exert little influence on the fragments. In the zygomatic arch region the pull of the masseter may cause downward displacement of the fragments. Normally such displacement is prevented by the temporal fascia which is attached to the superior surface of the zygomatic bone and arch and, in practice, displacement only occurs when this fascia is stripped from its attachments.

CHAPTER III

CLASSIFICATION

IN an area so anatomically complicated as the middle third of the facial skeleton, where fractures are usually comminuted, it is impossible to suggest a comprehensive classification which includes all possible bony injuries. The present knowledge of the lines of fracture produced in the middle third of the facial skeleton is based upon the experimental studies of fractures in this region carried out by Réné Le Fort in 1901. Following experimental trauma to the cadaver head and removal of the soft tissues, Le Fort discovered that the complex fracture patterns could be broadly subdivided into three groups:—

1. LE FORT I (low-level fracture).—The fracture line runs from the lateral margin of the anterior nasal aperture and passes laterally above the canine fossa, then below the zygomatic buttress and along the lateral antral wall and posteriorly across the pterygo-maxillary fissure to fracture the lower third of the pterygoid laminae. The fracture also passes along the lateral wall of the nose and joins the lateral fracture behind the tuberosity. This fracture may be unilateral or bilateral, and it causes detachment of the tooth-bearing portions of the upper jaw from the cranial base (*Fig. 5*).

2. LE FORT II (pyramidal or sub-zygomatic fracture).—This fracture runs from the thin middle area of the nasal bones down either side, across the frontal processes of the maxillae, across the lacrimal bones, and then downwards and forwards laterally crossing the inferior orbital margin in the region of the zygomatico-maxillary suture, down by the infra-orbital foramen and along the lateral wall of the antrum beneath the zygomatic buttress, across the pterygo-maxillary fissure to fracture the pterygoid laminae about half-way up.

3. LE FORT III (high-level or supra-zygomatic fracture).—The fracture commences near the frontonasal suture, the nasal bones, and lacrimal bones, runs across the thin orbital plates of the ethmoid, around the optic foramen and downwards laterally to the medial aspect of the posterior limit of the inferior orbital fissure. Then the fracture line descends across the upper posterior aspect of the maxillae, across the pterygo-maxillary fissure, and fractures the roots of the pterygoid laminae. A further line of fracture passes across the lateral wall of the orbit separating the zygomatic bone from the frontal bone. In this way the entire middle third of the facial skeleton becomes detached from the cranial base.

The Le Fort lines of fracture are most helpful in understanding the major fractures of the facial skeleton, but other fractures occur in this region.

A more exact classification (Rowe and Killey, 1968) is:—

A. FRACTURES NOT INVOLVING THE TEETH AND ALVEOLUS.—

1. *Central Region.*—

a. Fractures of nasal bones or septum.

b. Fractures of frontal process of the maxillae.

c. Fractures involving (*a*) and (*b*) which extend into the ethmoid.

2. *Lateral Region.*—Fractures of the zygomatic bone or arch.

a. First Degree: fracture of the arch or minimal displacement of the zygomatic bone.

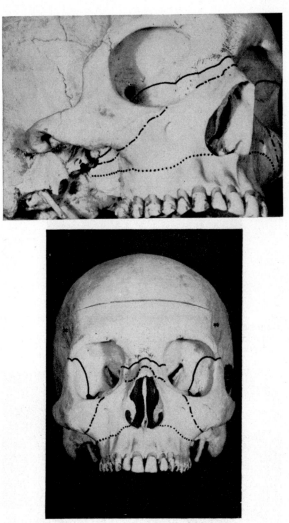

Fig. 5.—The Le Fort lines of fracture.

b. Second Degree: fracture of zygomatic bone and/or arch involving the lateral wall of the antrum and interfering with mandibular movement.

c. Third Degree: as above, with gross comminution of orbital floor and depression of the orbital level.

B. FRACTURES INVOLVING THE TEETH AND ALVEOLUS.—
1. *Central Region.*—
a. Alveolar fractures.
b. Low-level Le Fort I fractures.
c. Pyramidal Le Fort II fractures.

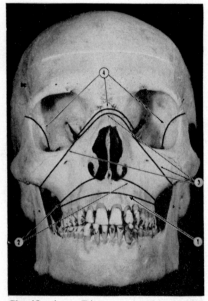

Fig. 6.—Classification. Diagram showing levels of fracture:
(1) Dento-alveolar; (2) Le Fort I, Guérin, or low-level; (3) Le Fort
II, pyramidal, or infra-zygomatic; (4) Le Fort III, high-level, or
supra-zygomatic.

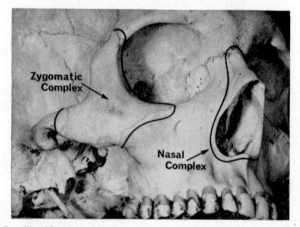

Fig. 7.—Classification. Nasal complex and zygomatic complex fractures.

2. *Combined Central and Lateral Fractures.*—
a. High-level supra-zygomatic fractures.
b. As type (*a*) with the addition of a midline split separating the maxillae into two.
c. As type (*a*) or (*b*), but associated with a fracture of the roof of the orbit or frontal bone.

This classification is comprehensive, but, for ordinary practical purposes in discussing signs and symptoms and planning treatment, a simple classification dividing the fractures into the six following categories is adequate and will be used in the ensuing text (*Figs.* 6, 7):—

1. Dento-alveolar fractures.
2. Zygomatic complex fractures.
3. Nasal complex fractures.
4. Le Fort I, Guérin, or low-level fractures.
5. Le Fort II, pyramidal, or infra-zygomatic fractures.
6. Le Fort III or supra-zygomatic fractures.

It should be remembered that, in the more severe injuries, several categories of fractures may coexist and the fractures may be unilateral or bilateral.

Table I.—ANALYSIS OF 629 MIDDLE THIRD FRACTURES
TO SHOW RELATIVE FREQUENCY

TYPE OF FRACTURE	NO. OF PATIENTS	PER CENT
Zygomatic bone and arch	336	53
Pre-maxilla	58	9·22
Unilateral Le Fort I	24	3·81
Unilateral Le Fort II	13	2·06
Le Fort I	27	4·29
Le Fort II	53	8·42
Le Fort I and II	36	5·73
Le Fort III	23	3·63
Le Fort I and III	12	1·9
Le Fort I, II, and III	3	0·47
Nasal fractures	44	6·99

RELATIVE FREQUENCY

Schuchardt and others (1966), with a total of 930 fractures involving the middle third, found 23·4 per cent were Le Fort II fractures, 18·5 per cent were Le Fort I fractures, 1·2 per cent were Le Fort III fractures, and 10·4 per cent were nasal fractures. The remainder were presumably dento-alveolar fractures. Rowe and Killey (1968) analysed 629 middle third fractures and the relative frequencies are shown in *Table I.* The relatively small number of nasal fractures probably does not represent the true incidence of this type of fracture, for they are not usually referred to a maxillo-facial unit.

CHAPTER IV

THE MANAGEMENT OF FRACTURES OF THE MIDDLE THIRD OF THE FACIAL SKELETON

IMMEDIATE TREATMENT

IN the period immediately following the accident, no treatment of the facial fracture is required unless it has a direct bearing upon the patency of the patient's airway or the control of haemorrhage. The definitive reduction and fixation of the facial fracture is never a life-saving measure, and the immediate treatment should be directed to the patient's general medical condition.

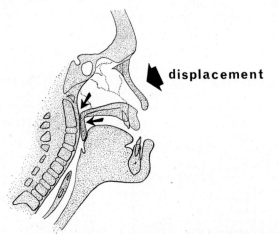

displacement

Fig. 8.—Bones of the middle third of the facial skeleton driven down the inclined plane shown in *Fig.* 2, p. 12. This occludes the oral airway.

The Airway.—First, the clinician should make certain that the patient s airway is adequate.

In Le Fort I, II, and III fractures, the upper jaw may have been pushed downwards and backwards so that the soft palate is resting upon the dorsum of the tongue and occludes the oral airway (*Fig.* 8). In such cases two fingers are inserted behind the hard palate and the upper jaw is pulled gently upwards and forwards to enable the patient to breathe through the mouth. Artificial oral airways, such as the Guedel pattern, are not well tolerated by patients with facial fractures and it is often time wasting to insert one.

The patient's lips should be liberally coated with sterile petroleum jelly to prevent them adhering together with blood-clot, and so interfering with respiration. This simple measure should be continued throughout treatment because it does much to ensure the comfort of the patient as well as facilitating oral respiration.

In Le Fort II and III fractures and with severe injuries to the nasal complex, the nares are blocked with blood-clot or are bleeding profusely; in either event there is occlusion of the nasal airway. The nose should be cleared with a suction apparatus and then a Magill's No. 3 flanged nasal tube is passed down each nostril. Any nasopharyngeal airway may be used, provided that a safety-pin is inserted at the external end to prevent it from slipping down the throat. The presence of a nasopharyngeal airway does not ensure maintenance of a clear airway because later it may become blocked with blood-clot and mucus or become kinked against the posterior

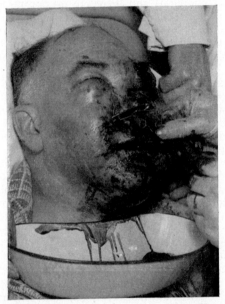

Fig. 9.—First-aid treatment of severe Le Fort III type injury. Note the two nasopharyngeal airways which are prevented from passing into the throat by safety-pins through the ends of the tubes. The nasopharyngeal airways are being kept patent by aspiration using a narrow tube attached to a suction apparatus.

pharyngeal wall. Constant supervision is necessary to confirm that the nasopharyngeal airway is patent, and this is done by frequent aspiration of the tubes, using a 1½-ft. or 45-cm. length of narrow bore ⅛-in. or 3-mm. diameter polythene tubing attached to the end of the sucker nozzle. Such an attachment is invaluable in the management of these fractures as it enables the pharynx to be aspirated through the nasopharyngeal airway and can also be used for sucking out the mouth (*Fig.* 9). The insertion of the nasopharyngeal airway is valuable also in controlling any epistaxis.

If the nasopharyngeal airway becomes kinked against the posterior pharyngeal wall, it should be pulled out for a short distance and the safety-pin adjusted to prevent it extending so far back. Sometimes it is sufficient to twist the tube round a little because only its orifice may be occluded against the posterior pharyngeal wall. Continuous supervision by the operator or by an experienced member of the nursing staff is necessary at this stage to ensure that the patient maintains a clear airway.

A careful examination of the oral cavity should be made in case dentures or portions of dentures are still in situ and these should be removed together with avulsed, loose, or broken teeth which are so mobile that there is a risk of their being inhaled.

The unconscious patient should be nursed on his side so that blood and saliva can run out of the oral and nasal cavities.

If the patient is conscious and there are no contra-indications, such as a fracture of the vertebrae, the patient should be nursed in a sitting position and the back rest and pillows should be arranged so that the chin is well forward and blood and saliva can dribble out of the mouth. This position is also comfortable for the patient and facilitates respiration.

The simple measures already mentioned are sufficient to ensure a patent airway, and it is unnecessary to perform a tracheostomy in the so-called 'civilian type' fracture of the middle third. Tracheostomy is, however, often required in patients who have sustained a so-called 'gun-shot' type injury—that is, a fracture of the middle third associated with a severe soft-tissue laceration and with soft- and hard-tissue loss.

Indications for Tracheostomy.—The indications for tracheostomy are gross retroposition of the middle third of the facial skeleton which is impacted and cannot be brought forwards by digital manipulation, severe oedema of the glottis, and uncontrollable post-nasal haemorrhage.

Haemorrhage.—The majority of fractures of the middle third of the facial skeleton are closed injuries, and, in spite of the extensive nature of the skeletal damage, severe haemorrhage is unusual. If there are associated soft-tissue lacerations, they may require urgent attention to control the haemorrhage, but, apart from an epistaxis and possibly some bleeding from lacerations in the alveolus, the average facial fracture does not bleed excessively and the control of haemorrhage presents no problem. Facial fractures associated with extensive damage to the soft tissues, as in the so-called gun-shot' type fractures, are frequently complicated by severe haemorrhage and will probably require transfusion. Blood must always be taken for cross matching. These cases are also liable to develop secondary haemorrhage.

Shock.—Shock is not usually a prominent feature of a fracture of the middle third of the facial skeleton, and if such a patient is severely shocked the possibility of the coexistence of some other more serious injury should be suspected.

PRELIMINARY EXAMINATION

After the operator has established a satisfactory airway and controlled possible haemorrhage, a full examination of the patient should be carried out. If the patient is unconscious or obviously severely ill, this should be limited to a few essential investigations and the more detailed examination should be left until the patient's general condition has improved.

The cranium should be inspected for evidence of lacerations and bony damage and the level of consciousness should be ascertained. The eyes should be examined for evidence of damage to the globe and the pupils should be inspected for variation in size and reaction to light. Special attention should be paid to the possibility of intracranial, intrathoracic, and intra-abdominal haemorrhage. The body should be inspected for evidence of fractures, especially of the cervical vertebrae. The possibility of damage to the kidneys, ureters, and urethra should be considered, and the first specimen of urine passed by the patient should be inspected and, if necessary, tested for blood.

If any serious associated injury is discovered, immediate treatment must be instituted, but if the operator is satisfied that the patient is in no immediate danger the case can be left until the general condition improves.

The nursing staff should be instructed to keep a half-hourly pulse chart and the blood-pressure should be recorded every hour. A fluid balance chart is begun and the pupils are inspected at intervals to note any variation in size. To prevent the development of infection in the fracture haematoma and in any associated soft-tissue injuries, the patient should be given intramuscular penicillin, one million units per day. Penicillin does not pass into the cerebrospinal fluid in adequate therapeutic concentrations, and as a prophylactic against meningitis if cerebrospinal fluid rhinorrhoea is present, the patient should be given a course of sulphonamide treatment. An initial dose of sulphadiazine, 2 g., is followed by 1 g. 6-hourly, the course to be continued for five days or longer if there is an established cerebrospinal fluid leak. If the patient is unconscious or unable to swallow, the sulphadiazine is given intramuscularly. If the patient can swallow, $\frac{1}{2}$ oz. or 15 ml. of Mist. Pot. Cit. should be given with each dose of sulphonamide, and an adequate amount of fluids should be given.

If the patient is on restricted fluids because of an associated head injury and has to have a protracted course of sulphonamides, it is advisable to examine the urine daily for evidence of crystals and red cells in case crystalluria is developing.

Pain.—Pain is not a prominent feature of fractures of the middle third of the facial skeleton, but patients frequently have cerebral irritation. The safest and most useful treatment for this condition is 3–8 ml. of paraldehyde intramuscularly.

Powerful analgesics and hypnotics should not be given in the early stages of treatment as they make the assessment of the level of consciousness more difficult.

Morphine is contra-indicated as it depresses the cough reflex, and so encourages the aspiration of blood into the trachea, and it also depresses the respiratory centre. Morphine also produces a miosis and so masks any pupillary changes which may be occurring as the result of an intracranial haemorrhage.

It is advisable to restrict the routine use of analgesics for patients with facial fractures. Once the fracture has been reduced and adequately immobilized, there should be no pain and the onset or persistence of pain is usually an indication that something is going wrong. This valuable symptom should not be masked with analgesics.

In the recent fracture where there is some difficulty with the airway, the use of powerful analgesics or hypnotics may possibly lead to the patient being suffocated during sleep, and therefore considerable caution should be exercised in the use of these drugs.

When this preliminary treatment has been carried out and the operator is satisfied that the patient is in no immediate danger, the patient can either be left until the general medical condition improves or a full general examination of the patient and local investigation of the facial injury can be carried out.

The reduction and fixation of a facial injury is never in itself an urgent procedure, and if there is doubt about the patient's general medical condition he should not be subjected to a general anaesthetic. Provided the patient is having antibiotic and sulphonamide therapy, the fracture will not become infected, and it is amazing how rapidly the patient's general condition will improve with even twenty-four hours' rest. The majority of the deaths in subjects suffering from maxillo-facial injuries occur as a result of ill patients being rushed to the operating theatre and subjected to a protracted operation.

If there are lacerations they should be sutured within twenty-four hours, and if it is intended to defer the operation these lacerations should be closed by suturing them under local analgesia.

General Medical Examination

As soon as the patient's medical condition permits, a detailed general medical examination should be carried out and then the facial fracture is investigated.

CHAPTER V

HISTORY AND LOCAL EXAMINATION

HISTORY OF THE INJURY AND DESCRIPTION OF THE PATIENT'S SYMPTOMS

IF THE patient is unconscious or confused, any relevant facts concerning the accident and the subsequent management of the patient must be obtained from eye-witnesses, ambulance men, or medical and dental practitioners who may have attended the patient following the injury.

If the patient is conscious and co-operative a history can be obtained, but as patients with facial injuries may experience some difficulty in talking owing to the pain and mobility of the fractures the interrogation should be brief at this stage.

It is prudent to ask if loss of consciousness has occurred and, in that event, whether the patient can remember up to the moment of the accident or whether there is a memory gap. Retrograde amnesia is failure to remember up to the time of injury and anterograde amnesia is loss of memory following the accident—both are indicative of cerebral damage.

It is also important to inquire whether the patient has any difficulty in breathing or swallowing and whether he has a headache or pain elsewhere in the body.

Information as to whether the patient was being treated with insulin, steroids, or anticoagulants prior to the accident is also most important.

A detailed history is obtained when the patient can talk more comfortably.

LOCAL CLINICAL EXAMINATION OF THE FACIAL INJURY

The examination of a patient with a recent severe injury to the middle third of the facial skeleton will be greatly facilitated if the patient's face is gently washed with warm water and cotton-wool swabs to remove caked blood. The congealed blood in the palate and buccal sulcus can be removed with cotton-wool held in untoothed forceps. Sometimes cotton-wool swabs dipped in hydrogen peroxide will facilitate the removal of any particularly tenacious clots in the mouth and upon the teeth. Care must be taken not to introduce hydrogen peroxide into a compound fracture owing to the risk of causing surgical emphysema or of introducing infection into the fracture line. After the blood has been cleaned away, the injury usually appears less severe.

On Inspection Externally.—The operator should take careful note of oedema, ecchymosis, and soft-tissue lacerations.

Any obvious bony deformities, haemorrhage, or cerebrospinal fluid leak should be recorded.

On Palpation.—Gentle palpation should begin at the back of the head and the cranium should be explored for wounds and bony injuries. Then the fingers should be run lightly over the zygomatic bones and arch, and around the rim of the orbits. Areas of tenderness, step deformities, and unnatural mobility are noted.

Next, the nasal complex is examined in the same manner.

The eyelids are gently separated and, if the patient is conscious, the vision is tested in each eye. Then the patient is asked to follow the clinician's finger with his eyes and asked to report if diplopia occurs. A note is made of alteration in the size of the two pupils, and the light reflex is tested. The extent of the subconjunctival ecchymosis is confirmed. Finally, the operator tests the two cheeks for anaesthesia in the distribution of the infra-orbital nerve.

On Inspection Intra-orally.—Gagging of the occlusion, derangement of the bite, lacerations, ecchymosis, and damage to the teeth and/or alveolus are noted.

On Palpation.—Areas of tenderness, bony irregularities, crepitus, and mobility of the teeth and the alveolus are noted.

Next, the tooth-bearing segment is gently manipulated to elicit unnatural mobility. A finger and thumb are then placed over the frontonasal suture line and movement of the facial skeleton is demonstrated by pressure from the fingers in the palate. A false impression of mobility of the middle third of the facial skeleton can be obtained, especially in the unconscious patient, by pressure in the palate alone, for the upper part of the head moves inside the epicranial aponeurosis producing the illusion of movement of the middle third of the facial skeleton. If the dento-alveolar segment moves independently of the remainder of the facial skeleton, it will be noted that an associated Le Fort I type of fracture is present. Next, the teeth are tapped and the 'cracked cup' sound is elicited if there is a fracture above the teeth. Finally, if the patient has teeth, they are examined with a mirror and probe to demonstrate possible fracture, mobility, and subluxation.

CHAPTER VI

CLINICAL FINDINGS IN THE VARIOUS
TYPES OF FRACTURE

A. DENTO-ALVEOLAR FRACTURES (SIGNS AND SYMPTOMS)

DENTO-ALVEOLAR injuries consist of fracture, subluxation, or avulsion of the teeth, with or without an associated fracture of the alveolus, and they may occur as a clinical entity or in conjunction with any other type of fracture.

Damage to the Teeth.—One of the most common fractures following an injury to the face is damage to the crown of a tooth, which may fracture with or without exposure of the pulp canal.

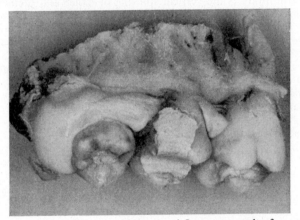

Fig. 10.—Dento-alveolar fracture of the antral floor as a result of an extraction accident.

Often the facial injury forces the soft tissues of the upper lip against the incisor teeth, producing a ragged laceration on the inner aspect of the upper lip and sometimes there is a full-thickness wound. Frequently, such an injury smashes the crown of one or more teeth, and portions of these crowns or even entire teeth become embedded in the upper lip.

Fractures of the roots of teeth also occur and sometimes such teeth are comminuted beneath the gum and frequently only an apex remains.

In an unconscious patient a fractured portion of tooth or a tooth which is completely avulsed may be inhaled at the time of the accident, and it is always advisable when a tooth or portion of tooth is missing following a facial injury to have a radiograph of the patient's chest, especially if there was loss of consciousness at the time of the accident.

Subluxation of one or more teeth without an associated fracture of the teeth leads to mobility and displacement of the teeth concerned with derangement of the occlusion.

Alveolar Fracture.—Fractures of the alveolus may occur with or without associated injuries of the teeth.

Fracture of the maxillary tuberosity and fracture of the antral floor are relatively common complications of exodontia. (*Fig.* 10.)

Facial injuries often produce multiple fractures of the alveolus and if the blow is especially violent there may be gross comminution of the alveolus, usually in the incisor area. If teeth were present, these too are usually comminuted, and often there is an extensive wound in the gingiva.

Clinical Examination.—There may be a full-thickness wound of the lip or, on gently lifting the upper lip, there may be a ragged laceration on its inner aspect. The lip is usually oedematous and there is ecchymosis.

On inspecting the teeth and gums there may be lacerations, ecchymosis, and obvious deformity of the alveolus. Where teeth have been knocked out there will be obvious extraction wounds and the remaining teeth may be mobile, subluxated, displaced, or fractured.

A common injury is the vertical splitting of molar and premolar teeth, caused when the lower teeth are forced against the occlusal surfaces of the upper teeth. At first sight such teeth appear normal, but on careful examination the extensive damage will be obvious and often a considerable number of teeth are involved.

A careful inspection of all teeth with a mirror and probe should always be carried out.

On Palpation.—The lip should be gently palpated and, if present, portions of teeth can usually be felt in the substance of the lip.

Gentle palpation of the alveolus will reveal bony deformity, and crepitus is felt if the alveolus is comminuted.

All teeth should be examined for mobility and split-type fractures, and finally the entire dento-alveolar segment should be tested to see whether it is detached from the remainder of the facial skeleton.

Fractures of teeth beneath the gum and the presence of apices can be detected only by intra-oral radiographs.

B. Fractures of the Zygomatic Complex

The zygomatic bone is intimately associated with the maxilla and frontal and temporal bones, and as they are usually involved when a zygomatic bone fracture occurs it is more accurate to refer to such injuries as 'zygomatic complex fractures'.

Some authors refer to the 'zygomatico-maxillary complex', but this description does not take account of the frontal and temporal bones.

The zygomatic bone usually fractures in the region of the zygomatico-frontal suture, the zygomatico-temporal suture, and the zygomatico-maxillary suture. It is unusual for the zygomatic bone itself to be fractured, but occasionally it may be split across and when there has been extreme violence the bone may even be comminuted. The zygomatic arch may be fractured without displacement of the zygomatic bone and in fractures involving the zygomatic bone the zygomatic arch may or may not be involved.

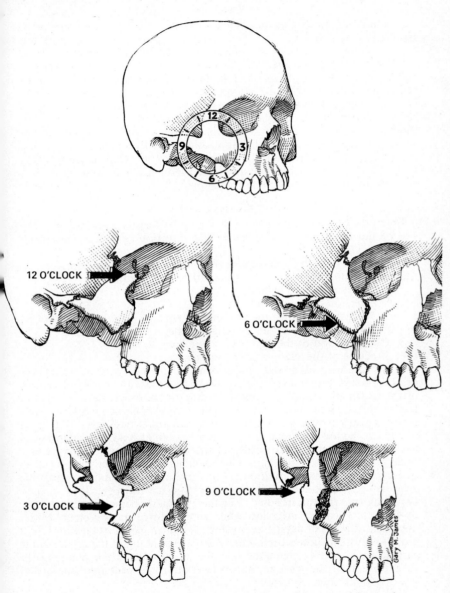

Fig. 11.—The main types of displacement in fractures of the zygomatic complex. If an imaginary clock face is superimposed over the body of the zygomatic bone, then force applied at 12 o'clock will result in inward displacement of the zygomatic bone with inversion of the orbital rim, while force at 6 o'clock will cause depression of the bone with eversion of the orbital rim. Force at 3 o'clock will cause depression with medial rotation and force at 9 o'clock depression with distal rotation.

Incidence

Fractures of the zygomatic complex occur as isolated fractures or in association with the Le Fort Type III fracture and they constitute the most common fracture of the middle third of the facial skeleton.

Kulowski (1956) analysed 295 facial fractures in which there were 62 middle third fractures, 22 of which involved the zygomatic bone. Maronneaud and others (1959), in 274 upper jaw fractures, found 164 zygomatic bone fractures. Donaldson (1961), in a series of 335 fractures, found 38 per cent involved the zygomatic bone. In 1966 Schuchardt and colleagues published a series of 2901 facial fractures and 22·2 per cent of the upper jaw fractures involved the zygomatic bone. Rowe and Killey (1968), in a series of 629 fractures of the middle third of the facial skeleton, found that 322, or 51·19 per cent, involved the zygomatic bone and 14, or 2·22 per cent, involved the zygomatic arch alone.

Classification

Fractures of the zygomatic complex may be classified according to the site of the fracture and the degree and direction of the displacement. (*Fig.* 11.) They are:—

1. Fracture of the zygomatic complex with minimal or no displacement.
2. Inward displacement of the zygomatic complex with:—
    a. Inversion of the orbital rim.
    b. Eversion of the orbital rim.
    c. Medial rotation of the zygomatic bone.
    d. Distal rotation of the zygomatic bone.
3. Comminution of the zygomatic complex.
4. Fracture of the zygomatic arch alone.

In all fractures other than those confined to the zygomatic arch, the orbital floor is comminuted to a greater or lesser extent. The displacement of the zygomatic complex varies according to the exact site of impact of the fracturing force. Force over the area of the zygomatico-frontal process tends to result in depression with inversion of the orbital rim, while force applied at the lower border of the zygomatic bone could cause depression and eversion of the lower border of the orbit. Force on the zygomatic bone in the region of the zygomatico-maxillary suture line may result in depression with medial rotation, while force applied distally towards the zygomatic arch could cause depression with distal rotation. If an imaginary clock face is superimposed over the zygomatic bone, maximum force at 12 o'clock causes inversion while similar force at 6 o'clock causes eversion. A point of impact at 3 o'clock results in medial rotation while at 9 o'clock distal rotation can occur. An understanding of the nature of the displacement of the zygomatic complex is of value when planning the disimpaction of the fracture and in evaluating the probable stability of the fragments after reduction.

Signs and Symptoms

The signs and symptoms of a fracture of the zygomatic bone are closely related to the surgical anatomy of the part.

On Inspection.—When the zygomatic bone is fractured near the zygomatico-frontal, zygomatico-temporal, and zygomatico-maxillary sutures, it is displaced inwards to a greater or lesser extent. There may be minimal displacement or an obvious unsightly flattening of one cheek bone may occur.

The amount of depression may be masked if the patient normally has a rather fat face; on the other hand, ethnic types, such as the Slavonic race, who normally have prominent cheek bones, may exhibit marked flattening of the face with only moderate inward displacement of the zygomatic bone.

The physical sign of flattening of the cheek bone is best seen by viewing the patient either from above by standing behind and above the patient and comparing the two sides of the face, or by viewing the two cheek bones from below. Flattening should be looked for immediately after the accident before the area is masked by oedema or after the swelling has subsided.

The speed with which oedema occurs varies considerably. In some thin, elderly patients, flattening may be obvious up to about an hour after the injury; on the other hand, young, plump-faced individuals swell up almost immediately. It is usually possible to palpate the zygoma and if oedema is masking the flattening, the forefingers should be placed on the zygomatic bones on each side and the relative position of the two fingers can then be compared. Even with marked oedema this manœuvre enables an assessment to be made of the degree of flattening. Most of the overlying swelling subsides in about a week, but the full extent of the flattening is not apparent until all oedema has completely disappeared, which takes up to three weeks.

Circumorbital ecchymosis occurs in all cases of zygomatic bone fractures. The ecchymosis develops within a short time of the injury and the bruising is of more or less uniform intensity and is limited by the attachments of the orbicularis oculi. It is usually more marked in elderly patients who often bruise more readily. It can be distinguished from a 'black eye' by the fact that there is a generalized swelling with more or less uniform intensity of the ecchymosis, whereas in the black eye the oedema is often localized, usually beneath the eye, and the ecchymosis is patchy and of varying intensity. The differential diagnosis between fracture of the zygomatic bone and a 'black eye' can, of course, be confirmed by the presence or absence of subconjunctival ecchymosis. In zygomatic bone fractures, the haemorrhage beneath the conjunctiva occupies the outer quadrant of the eye unless there is an associated fracture in the region of the nasal bones or frontal process of the maxilla when the inner quadrant of the eye will also be involved. There is no limit posteriorly to the subconjunctival ecchymosis and this can be demonstrated by asking the patient to look inwards, when the ecchymosis will be seen to extend posteriorly into the orbit.

It is possible to have subconjunctival ecchymosis with a 'black eye', but the ecchymosis is patchy and does not form a continuous sheet as with fracture of the zygomatic bone. Subconjunctival ecchymosis lasts about a month or six weeks and gradually disappears. Unlike bruising elsewhere in the body, the ecchymosis stays a bright red colour as oxygen can pass through the conjunctiva and oxygenate the haemoglobin in the red blood-corpuscles.

As the zygomatic bone is displaced into the maxillary sinus in the region of the zygomatico-maxillary suture, the outer wall of the antrum is comminuted and the antrum fills with blood. This can be seen on X-ray examination as an opacity of the antrum, and at the time of injury and for a short time afterwards the blood escapes from the antrum through the ostium into the nose and produces a unilateral epistaxis.

If the fracture involves the infra-orbital nerve, it may lead to either a neurapraxia or a neurotmesis of the nerve. The patient complains of anaesthesia of the cheek and side of the nose, and, depending on the degree of damage to the nerve, this anaesthesia may persist for eight to eighteen months but eventually disappears completely.

As the zygomatic bone is displaced inwards, it may impinge on the coronoid process and interfere with mandibular movements. If the mandible is widely open at the time of injury, the zygomatic bone may be driven in to such an extent that it is impossible for the patient to close the mouth.

If the mouth was closed at the time of injury, the patient may be unable to open the mouth.

In all cases lateral excursion of the mandible to the fractured side is impaired and usually the patient will be unable to protrude the mandible.

If the fracture involves any of the extra-ocular muscles or the nerves supplying these muscles, the patient will have diplopia. This is a common symptom in the early stages of the injury, and is often caused by oedema and effusion in the region of the extra-ocular muscles. This type of diplopia is temporary, but that due to damage to extra-ocular muscles or their nerves is, of course, much more serious.

Temporary diplopia is due to oedema and haemorrhage in and around the orbital muscles. Barclay (1960) reviewed 383 fractures of the zygomatic complex and found an incidence of 8·4 per cent cases of diplopia. Mansfield (1948), in 153 cases, found that 13·1 per cent had diplopia. Barclay (1960) found 10 per cent of patients had diplopia, half of which were transient.

Testing the ocular movements by having the patient follow a moving finger held before his eyes will enable the operator to decide which muscles are involved.

Another troublesome cause of diplopia is enophthalmos. This occurs in severe fractures of the zygomatic bone when the orbital floor is comminuted. When this happens, the periorbital fat herniates into the maxillary antrum and if the condition is not treated an enophthalmos results.

Alteration of the level of the eye without interference with the extra-ocular muscles and their nerve-supply does not cause diplopia. Anyone can demonstrate this fact by turning the head on one side so that one eye is lower than the other.

It is not unusual to find a patient with one eye considerably lower than the other, who does not complain of diplopia. Alteration in the ocular level in patients with fracture of the zygomatic bone depends on the level at which the fracture occurs in the region of the zygomatico-frontal suture.

The globe of the eye is supported by Lockwood's suspensory ligament. This is a fascial sling which is attached in the region of the lacrimal bone and is inserted into Whitnall's tubercle on the inner aspects of the zygomatic bone just beneath the zygomatico-frontal suture.

If the fracture occurs beneath Whitnall's tubercle the zygomatic bone can be grossly displaced downwards without alteration in the level of the globe of the eye. However, if the fracture occurs above Whitnall's tubercle, the globe is displaced downwards with the zygomatic bone. When the globe of the eye is displaced downwards the upper lid follows it and produces a characteristic 'hooding' of the globe. This physical sign is especially obvious when the oedema in the area has subsided.

Sometimes, as the zygomatic bone is driven in, the entire maxilla is 'sprung' down without being fractured and there may be temporary gagging of the occlusion in the molar area on the fractured side.

Comminution of the outer walls of the maxillary antrum may damage the anterior, middle, or posterior superior dental nerves, with resulting anaesthesia of the teeth and gums.

Intra-orally there is often marked ecchymosis in the upper buccal sulcus in the region of the zygomatic buttress.

On Palpation.—There is tenderness over the zygomatic bone, often with an obvious step deformity in the orbital rim in the region of the zygomatico-maxillary suture.

There is also tenderness on palpation over the zygomatic buttress area intra-orally, and sometimes crepitus may be felt.

Summary of Symptoms.—The patient may complain of:—
1. Flattening of cheek.
2. Swelling and bruising around the eye.
3. Blood-shot eye.
4. Double vision.
5. Squint.
6. One eye too far back.
7. One eye lower than the other.
8. Tenderness over the cheek.
9. Anaesthesia of the cheek and gums.
10. Lump on the lower orbital rim.
11. Difficulty in either opening or closing the mouth.
12. Inability to move the jaw towards the injured side.
13. Gagging of the back teeth on the injured side.

Summary of Physical Signs.—
On inspection externally:
1. Circumorbital ecchymosis.
2. Subconjunctival ecchymosis.
3. Oedema of cheek.
4. Flattening in region of zygoma on injured side.
5. Limitation of ocular movements.
6. Diplopia.
7. Strabismus.
8. Enophthalmos.
9. Limitation of lateral excursion of mandible to injured side.
10. Limitation of opening or closing of mandible.
11. Unilateral epistaxis on injured side.

On palpation:
1. Tenderness over cheek bone.
2. Notch in lower rim of orbit in the region of the zygomatico-maxillary suture.
3. Anaesthesia of the cheek.

On inspection intra-orally:
1. Ecchymosis in upper buccal sulcus in region of zygomatic buttress.
2. Possible gagging of occlusion in molar area on injured side.

On palpation:
1. Tenderness in upper buccal sulcus in region of zygomatic buttress.
2. Anaesthesia of upper gum.

Fractures of the Zygomatic Arch.—Fractures of the zygomatic arch may coexist with fractures of the zygomatic bone. In such cases, the distinguishing features of the zygomatic arch fractures are obscured by the more gross physical signs associated with the zygomatic bone fractures.

Fractures of the zygomatic arch tend to impinge on the coronoid process and so extreme interference with mandibular movements may be found in combined zygomatic bone and zygomatic arch fractures.

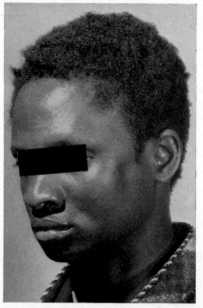

Fig. 12.—Clinical photograph showing typical circular depression seen over the zygomatic arch in an isolated zygomatic arch fracture with V type displacement.

The zygomatic arch may be fractured without fracturing the zygomatic bone at its zygomatico-frontal and zygomatico-maxillary suture lines. In such a condition the only visible evidence of fracture is a depression of about 1 in. or 2·5 cm. in diameter over the zygomatic arch associated with limitation of mandibular excursion to the injured side and possible interference with mandibular opening or closing.

The depression is obvious immediately after fracture of the arch, but it often becomes obscured by oedema shortly after injury only to become visible again when the swelling subsides in about a week. (*Fig.* 12.)

No other physical signs and symptoms typical of a fracture of the zygomatic bone are present.

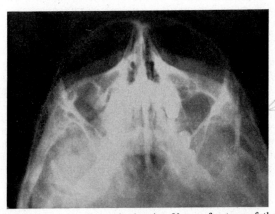

Fig. 13.—Occipito-mental radiograph showing V type fracture of the zygomatic arch.

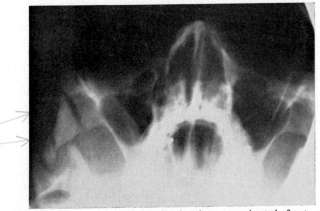

Fig. 14.—Occipito-mental radiograph showing comminuted fracture of the zygomatic arch.

Isolated fractures of the zygomatic arch are uncommon. In Donaldson's (1961) series of facial fractures 3 per cent involved the zygomatic arch and in 336 fractures of the zygomatic complex (Rowe and Killey, 1968) only 14 were confined to the zygomatic arch. Knight and North (1961) found 10 per cent zygomatic arch fractures in their 120 cases of zygomatic complex fractures.

Fractures of the zygomatic arch can be divided into two main varieties:—

1. The triple fracture of the arch with a depressed V type of displacement.

2. Comminution of the arch. (*Figs.* 13, 14.)

In the V type of displacement the apex of the V may impinge on the coronoid process and impede mandibular movements, especially lateral excursion to the injured side. In the absence of surgical correction this depression persists and constitutes a cosmetic deformity.

When the zygomatic arch is comminuted, the fragments usually reposition themselves presumably as a result of movements of the temporalis muscle and coronoid process beneath them. When the fragments are realigned they are held in position by the attachment of the temporalis fascia on their superior border. Fragments of the zygomatic arch are only displaced downwards if their attachment to the temporalis fascia is stripped away. In such a case transosseous wiring is required to immobilize the fragments. In all other cases the fascial attachments provide the necessary immobilization. Fractures of the zygomatic arch associated with fractures of the zygomatic bone and other elements of the zygomatic complex usually become repositioned when the main zygomatic bone fragment is surgically elevated into its correct position.

C. Isolated Orbital Floor Fractures

Applied Surgical Anatomy.—The orbit is said to be roughly pyramidal in shape with its apex at the optic foramen, but as the junctions between its alleged walls are rounded it does in fact resemble a cone. It has a medial and lateral surface, a roof and a floor. The wall on its medial aspect is thin and beneath it lie the ethmoidal air cells. Both the lateral wall and the roof are relatively thick, but the floor of the orbit which slopes upwards towards the optic foramen is extremely thin, particularly in the region of the infra-orbital groove which anteriorly becomes the infra-orbital canal.

The orbital floor is made up of the orbital portion of the maxillary bone and part of the zygomatic bone. It is bounded laterally by the inferior orbital fissure, posteriorly it is made up of the orbital process of the palatine bone and a small portion of the ethmoid bone. Medially the floor is bounded by the lacrimal bone.

The eyeball normally protrudes slightly beyond the orbital rim and it is suspended by Lockwood's ligament which runs from Whitnall's tubercle just below the zygomatico-frontal suture to the inner wall of the orbital rim. The eyeball itself is relatively tough and it is filled with incompressible vitreous humour. The remainder of the orbital cavity is filled with fat. A blow from an object of greater diameter than the orbital rim will force the eyeball back and as the orbit is more or less cone-shaped the orbital contents will be compressed. This raises the intra-orbital pressure and exerts a fracturing force, especially over the thin infra-orbital canal area and to a slightly lesser extent in the region of the ethmoid air cells. The walls of the orbit will therefore tend to fracture in these areas.

This type of injury has been called the 'orbital blow-out fracture'. However, it is possible to have a 'blow-in' fracture (Dingman and Natvig, 1964). This rare injury usually occurs in children when the bone is resilient and it is caused by trauma to the orbital rim which results in an inward buckling of the orbital floor. It is therefore more exact to describe all such injuries as 'isolated' orbital floor fractures.

In fractures caused by the blow-out mechanism the fragments are displaced downwards into the maxillary sinus and these bone particles sometimes remain attached to the periosteum or they may be completely detached and fall to the floor of the maxillary sinus. The peri-orbital fat prolapses into the maxillary sinus and if not replaced surgically this will lead to a residual enophthalmos.

The inferior rectus and inferior oblique muscles, which share a common fascial sheath, may become involved in the defect of the orbital floor or they can be bound down by subsequent fibrous tissue formation. Mechanical interference of this nature will prevent upward and outward rotation of the eye by the action of the inferior oblique muscle and upward rotation of the globe by inhibiting the unaided action of the superior rectus. This results in vertical diplopia with the false image above the true image which occurs when the patient looks upwards. Downward movement of the eye may be prevented by absence of inferior rectus activity. Damage to the nerves supplying these muscles may also occur. Fractures of the orbit can also be sustained as an extension of fractures of the zygomatic bone.

The mechanism of the blow-out fracture was demonstrated by Smith and Regan (1957). A hard ball was placed over the closed lids of the orbit of a cadaver, the hypotony of the globe being first increased to normal by an intravitreal injection of normal saline. The ball was then hit with a hammer. Dissection showed a comminuted floor of the orbit, but the orbital rim and zygomatic arch were intact.

Next, the orbit was exenterated and the ball replaced over the orbital rim. Repeated blows failed to produce comminution of the orbital floor. Extensive force, however, resulted in fracture of the orbital rim together with the orbital floor.

Signs and Symptoms.—In the immediate post-traumatic phase the characteristic signs and symptoms which are seen in the late stage of the untreated case are masked by oedema and ecchymosis, both within and external to the orbit. There is circumorbital and subconjunctival ecchymosis and sometimes marked surgical emphysema of the lids occurs due to the communication with the paranasal air sinuses. Fracture of the lamina papyracea is probably the site of the air leak and this condition usually occurs when the patient blows his nose violently. Unilateral epistaxis and paraesthesia of the infra-orbital nerve occur. There may be proptosis and there is limitation of vertical oculo-rotatory movement. This gives rise to diplopia on looking upwards with the false image above the true image. When the extravasated blood and tissue fluids subside enophthalmos occurs due to loss of peri-orbital fat into the maxillary sinus. Restriction of upward movement of the eye becomes more pronounced. Failure of upward rotation may also be due to damage to the superior rectus or its nerve supply. The differential diagnosis from entrapment of the inferior oblique muscle is made by the forced duction test.

Under local analgesia fine-toothed dissecting forceps are inserted under the globe of the eye to grasp the conjunctiva and subconjunctival tissues near the limbus just inferiorly to the cornea, and the globe is forcibly elevated. The two eyes are compared and an increased resistance is virtually diagnostic of a blow-out fracture with incarcerated orbital tissue.

Radiology.—The characteristic feature of the isolated orbital floor fracture is the absence of obvious bony damage to the zygomatic bone and arch even though clinical examination suggests the presence of such an injury. On routine views, however, there is an opacity of the maxillary sinus and the ethmoidal sinuses may also be cloudy due to fracture of the overlying bone and presence of blood in the air cells. Cramer et al. (1965) first described the so-called 'hanging drop' sign in standard sinus views. This opacity consists of a smooth convexity which faces downwards, suspended from the roof of the maxillary sinus, and is made up of extravasated blood. In view of the fact that isolated orbital floor fractures cannot be diagnosed with certainty from routine radiographic views, it is essential to have tomograms of the area in all cases of suspected orbital floor fractures. Milauskas (1969) advocates the use of orbitography by injecting hypaque into the extraconal space in order to demonstrate this fracture.

D. Fractures of the Nasal Complex

Surgical Anatomy.—It is possible for the nasal bones alone to be fractured, but it is more usual for there to be an associated fracture of the frontal processes of the maxillae which articulate with the nasal bones on their lateral aspect.

In a very severe fracture the lower part of the lateral wall of the orbit may be involved, with associated fractures of the lacrimal bone and the orbital laminae of the ethmoid.

Fractures of the nasal region usually involve the nasal septum. Sometimes the septal cartilage is merely dislodged from its groove in the vomer, but in more serious injuries the vomer and perpendicular and cribriform plates of the ethmoid may be fractured. Very severe injuries of this kind may give rise to a cerebrospinal fluid rhinorrhoea.

The displacement of the fragments depends on the direction of the fracturing force. Force applied laterally to the nose leads to the nasal bones and associated portions of the frontal processes of the maxillae being displaced to one side. (*Fig.* 15.) At the same time, the septal cartilage which is attached to the inner aspect of the nasal bones is subjected to a strain which causes it to be detached from its groove in the vomer. More violent force will, of course, lead to comminution of the vomer together with the perpendicular and possibly cribriform plates of the ethmoid.

Force applied anteriorly over the bridge of the nose leads to the nasal bones being driven inwards, while the frontal processes of the maxillae fracture and are splayed outwards. (*Fig.* 16.) This leads to a flattened, depressed nose, and again the underlying septal cartilage and the vomer and perpendicular and cribriform plates of the ethmoid may be involved.

If untreated, the lateral type of injury will result in a deviation of the nose to one side, with probably a blockage of both nares.

Untreated anterior-type injuries leave a flattened nose with thickened bridge which is especially ugly if the lacrimal bones and orbital laminae of the ethmoid bones are involved. This leads to an increase in distance between the inner canthi, and creates the illusion that there is an increased separation of the eyes.

Signs and Symptoms of Fractures of the Nasal Complex.—

On Inspection: In the recent injury much of the skeletal displacement will be masked by the overlying oedema.

There will be bilateral circumorbital ecchymosis, more marked on the medial aspect opposite the nose. There will be subconjunctival ecchymosis mainly confined to the medial half of the eyes. The entire nose may be

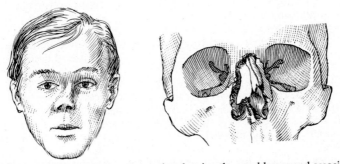

Fig. 15.—Fracture of the nasal complex showing the nasal bones and associated portions of the frontal process of the maxilla driven laterally as a result of force applied to one side of the nose.

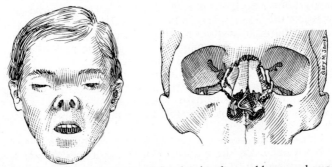

Fig. 16.—Fracture of the nasal complex showing the nasal bones and associated portions of the frontal process of the maxilla driven inwards as a result of force sustained over the bridge of the nose.

seen to be deviated to one side following a lateral injury while an anterior fracturing force produces a saddle-type depression of the bridge.

There is invariably epistaxis in both nostrils in the recent injury, and when the blood has clotted there may be a discharge of clear serum. If the cribriform plate of the ethmoid has been comminuted, there may be a cerebrospinal fluid leak. This cerebrospinal fluid may pass backwards down the throat and the patient will complain of a salty taste. The tissue over the bridge of the nose is thin and often the fragments of nasal bone penetrate the skin, rendering the fracture compound. If the tip of the nose is gently raised, it may be possible to see that the tip of the nasal septal cartilage is displaced. It should be remembered that many patients normally have deformity of the bony skeleton of the nose and/or an associated nasal septal defect, and a difficult diagnostic problem arises when a patient with a damaged nose sustains further trauma to that area.

On Palpation: On gentle palpation the underlying nasal bones may be felt to be mobile and comminuted. Often sharp step-defects in the nasal skeleton are felt. The area is acutely tender on palpation. Palpation is less painful over an old nasal fracture which has received further trauma without additional fracture.

When the naso-ethmoidal region has sustained considerable violence, as in Le Fort II or III type fractures, and is severely comminuted, the entire area gives the sensation of lead shot under the palpating finger.

E. Le Fort I, Low-level, or Guérin Type Fractures

This type of fracture may occur as a single clinical entity or in conjunction with Le Fort II or Le Fort III type fractures.

If it occurs as part of a more severe fracture its distinctive clinical appearance is largely masked by the associated Le Fort II or III type fracture.

If only a Le Fort I, low-level, or Guérin fracture is present, the signs and symptoms are as follows:—

On Inspection: In the recent injury, there may be slight swelling in the region of the upper lip, but there is no massive oedema of the tissues covering the middle third of the facial skeleton which produces the classic 'ballooning' of the facies in the Le Fort II and III type fractures. There is no circumorbital ecchymosis, no subconjunctival ecchymosis, no anaesthesia of the cheek, no flattening of the zygomatic region, and no disorganization of the naso-ethmoidal complex area.

Frequently, this type of fracture is caused by a blow with a sharp object in the front of the mouth above the apices of the teeth, and when this happens there is often a soft-tissue laceration in this area. Under these circumstances it is sometimes possible to see into the nares and the antra through the upper lip.

The dento-alveolar portion of the upper jaw is completely mobile and the patient usually has the mouth open to accommodate the fragment which has dropped on to the lower teeth.

Intra-orally: The entire tooth-bearing portion of the upper jaw is seen to be mobile. Usually there is marked deviation of the upper midline and one side of the upper jaw with its attached teeth is dropped lower than the other.

There is ecchymosis in the buccal sulcus, and probably an associated laceration.

On Palpation: The entire dento-alveolar portion of the upper jaw is found to be extremely mobile, and in the recent injury it can usually be repositioned with little difficulty into its correct anatomical situation.

Percussion of the upper teeth produces a distinctive 'cracked cup' sound similar to that produced when cracked china is tapped with a spoon.

All possible variations of open and closed type fractures may occur and it is possible to see the condition unilaterally when it involves only one maxilla, the tooth-bearing portion being split up the median palatal suture. The Le Fort I fracture may also be produced with a midline separation along the palate so that both fragments are mobile, and it may be complicated by subluxation or other damage to the associated teeth.

Le Fort I, low-level, or Guérin type fractures with the most spectacular downward displacement are often those associated with Le Fort II or III type fractures. In these cases the patient frequently complains of trismus or inability to open the mouth. The mandible is, however, already widely open, and by putting two fingers under the upper teeth and without an anaesthetic it is possible to lift up the dento-alveolar portion about 2 inches. Such injuries are often descriptively referred to as 'floaters' or 'loose faces'.

Sometimes a low-level fracture occurs with minimal displacement and the patient presents with a slight derangement of the occlusion and usually a deviation of the upper midline to one side or the other. Careful radiological examination is necessary to diagnose this type of injury, especially if there has been a time lag of several days before the patient is examined because this type of fracture unites very rapidly.

F. AND G. LE FORT II AND III TYPE FRACTURES
(SIGNS AND SYMPTOMS)

The signs and symptoms of the Le Fort II, or pyramidal, and the Le Fort III, or supra-zygomatic, type fractures appear similar on superficial examination. At first sight patients with either of these varieties of fracture are seen to have gross oedema of the tissues of the middle third of the facial skeleton, bilateral circumorbital ecchymosis and subconjunctival ecchymosis, derangement of the naso-ethmoidal complex, anaesthesia of the cheeks, and backward and downward displacement of the upper jaw (*Fig.* 17).

A more detailed clinical examination soon enables the clinician to distinguish between the two varieties.

F. LE FORT II OR PYRAMIDAL TYPE FRACTURE (SIGNS AND SYMPTOMS).—

In contradistinction to the Le Fort I type fracture, there is gross ballooning of the facies due to massive oedema of the tissues covering the middle third of the facial skeleton. This oedema develops very rapidly following the injury and is well established within minutes of the fracture occurring.

Bilateral circumorbital ecchymosis also develops almost immediately. The oedema around the eyes is often so marked that it is impossible to separate the lids to examine the globe. However, the eyes must be examined to exclude the possibility of serious injury to the globe which may require urgent treatment, and this is usually carried out by inserting retractors beneath the lids.

Subconjunctival ecchymosis usually develops rapidly, but it sometimes requires several hours to become fully established. The subconjunctival ecchymosis may extend over the outer and inner quadrants of the eye as the frontal process of the maxilla and nasal complex are usually involved, and there is usually some springing of the zygomatic bone at the time of the injury.

Sometimes the subconjunctival ecchymosis causes the conjunctiva to bulge, and when the circumorbital oedema subsides a little the conjunctiva is seen to herniate from beneath the lids. Occasionally, the zygomatic bones are not involved and then there is no subconjunctival ecchymosis in the outer quadrants.

In the early stage of the injury it is often difficult to test ocular movements or test for diplopia, but diplopia is usually present and ocular movements may be limited.

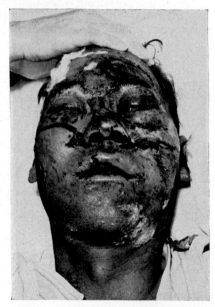

Fig. 17.—Le Fort III type fracture. Note ballooning of the facies and marked disorganization of the nasal complex. The nasal bridge has been pushed back.

Enophthalmos due to comminution of the orbital floor and herniation of the periorbital fat into the maxillary sinus is also difficult to demonstrate in the early stage of the injury. It is, fortunately, extremely rare for the fracturing force to damage the optic nerve as the nerve is protected by a strong ring of compact bone which forms the optic foramen and the fracture line goes round the foramen rather than through it. But, because it is possible for the sight to be impaired as a result of the injury, the patient's vision should be tested as soon as possible. It is difficult to detect an alteration of the pupillary level in the recently injured patient, but a careful examination at a later stage may elicit this physical sign. Careful note should be made of any variation in the size of the pupils on either side because a dilating pupil may be an early sign of intracranial haemorrhage.

As the fracture forces the bones of the middle third of the facial skeleton down the inclined plane formed by the frontal bone and the body of the sphenoid, the mandible is forced open and there is gagging of the molar teeth and retroposition of the upper incisors. This leads to considerable lengthening of the face, but this physical sign is masked by the oedema of the tissues of the face and is only noticeable when the oedema has subsided.

The naso-ethmoidal complex is disorganized and the nose is obviously broken, either being displaced to one side or with the bridge pushed in, producing a similar effect to turning a book inside out. There is also obvious lengthening of the nose due to the face having fallen. Blood and possibly cerebrospinal fluid trickle out of the nostrils, which are usually blocked by blood-clot.

On Palpation.—Gentle palpation of the zygomatic arch and zygomatic bone will confirm that neither of these structures is fractured, but it will reveal a notch in the lower border of the orbit on each side. It will also detect crepitus in the nasal complex as the nasal bones and frontal processes of the maxillae are usually comminuted.

The Le Fort II type fractures exhibit varying degrees of mobility of the main fragments. Sometimes the fractured portion is impacted and immobile on palpation, but at other times it is possible to place a thumb and finger over the region of the frontonasal suture and, with two fingers pressing in the palate, detect movement of the pyramidal-shaped block of bone. If there is an associated Le Fort I type fracture, it will be possible to move the dento-alveolar portion of the middle third independently. No movement of the zygomatic bone will be detected.

Tapping of the upper teeth will give a characteristic 'cracked cup' sound.

Summary of Symptoms.—
1. Swelling of face.
2. Swelling and bruising around both eyes.
3. Blood-shot eyes.
4. Pain over nose and face.
5. Deformity of nose.
6. Flattening of the middle of the face.
7. Difficulty in opening the mouth.
8. Inability to move the lower jaw.
9. Gagging of the back teeth.
10. Front teeth not meeting.
11. Bleeding from the nose and possibly salty fluid running down the nose or back of the throat.
12. Upper jaw seems to move.
13. Double vision.

Summary of Physical Signs.—
1. Gross oedema of the soft tissues over the middle third of the facial skeleton.
2. Bilateral circumorbital ecchymosis.
3. Bilateral subconjunctival ecchymosis, which may be confined to the inner half of the eye.
4. Obvious deformity of the nose.

5. Flattening of the middle of the face without corresponding flattening of the cheek bones.

6. Lengthening of the face.

7. Retroposition of the upper incisors.

8. Gagging of occlusion in the molar area.

9. Anterior open bite.

10. Soft palate depressed on to the dorsum of the tongue.

11. No tenderness over or disorganization and mobility of zygomatic bones and arch.

12. Possibly enophthalmos, diplopia, and limitation of ocular movements.

13. Sometimes no anaesthesia of the cheeks.

14. Mobility of a pyramidal area of the middle of the face, which can be demonstrated by bimanual palpation between the palate and the frontonasal suture.

15. Epistaxis.

16. Possibly a cerebrospinal fluid rhinorrhoea.

17. 'Cracked cup' sound on tapping teeth.

G. LE FORT III, HIGH-LEVEL, OR SUPRA-ZYGOMATIC FRACTURES (SIGNS AND SYMPTOMS).—Superficially, the Le Fort III fracture appears very similar to the Le Fort II type fracture, but it is usually obvious that the injury is very much more severe.

On Inspection Extra-orally.—In the recent injury there is massive oedema of the tissues of the middle third of the facial skeleton which produces the classic ballooning of the facies. Bilateral circumorbital ecchymosis is present and, when the lids are separated, extensive subconjunctival ecchymosis is present, often involving all quadrants. Often the conjunctiva bulges with the haematoma.

There may be strabismus, enophthalmos, diplopia, and limitation of ocular movements.

There is obvious disorganization of the nasal complex and the nose may either be pushed in or displaced to one side. There is obvious lengthening of the bridge of the nose due to the face dropping. The nares are almost blocked with blood-clot, and blood, serum, or cerebrospinal fluid may be seen escaping from the nostrils.

There is great lengthening of the face, but this is usually masked by the gross oedema of the soft tissues. When the swelling subsides in about a week or ten days, this lengthening of the face becomes very obvious. The excessive length of the bridge of the nose is especially noticeable at this stage. In this type of fracture there is often a dropping of the ocular level due to the fracture passing above Whitnall's tubercle and so removing the support of Lockwood's suspensory ligament. As one or both eyes drop, the upper lid follows the globe down, producing unilateral or bilateral 'hooding' of the eyes. This physical sign is specially obvious in the untreated fracture when the oedema has subsided completely. Flattening of one or both zygomatic bones may be seen, but here again, the swelling present in the recently injured patient may obscure the deformity which becomes more obvious as the oedema subsides.

On Palpation.—Gentle palpation over the zygomatic bones and zygomatic arch reveals areas of tenderness and step-deformities over the sites of fracture. If the bones are comminuted, crepitus is detected. By placing the finger-tips over the zygomatic bones bilaterally, some assessment of the displacement can be obtained by comparing the levels of the finger-tips, even though considerable oedema is present.

Gentle palpation of the nasal complex will reveal marked disruption of the bony structures with crepitus. Often in the closed injury the comminution feels like lead shot underneath the fingers.

If two fingers are placed over the frontonasal suture region and the dento-alveolar portion of the upper jaw is grasped with the other hand gentle movement of the entire face can be demonstrated. Often the zygomatic bones are mobile, independent of the rest of the facial skeleton.

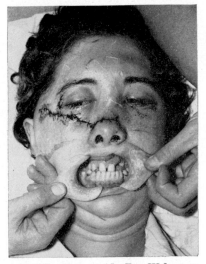

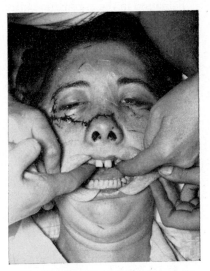

Fig. 18.—Untreated Le Fort III fracture two weeks after injury. Note backward displacement of upper teeth. Patient complained of being unable to open her mouth. The mandible was, in fact, widely open, due to the upper jaw having dropped.

Fig. 19.—Gentle upward manipulation of the upper tooth-bearing segment demonstrates extent to which upper jaw had dropped in patient shown in *Fig.* 18.

Frequently, in the Le Fort III type fracture coexistent Le Fort I and Le Fort II fractures occur and by gentle palpation of the fragments this fact can be demonstrated quite easily.

Usually both cheeks are anaesthetic owing to involvement of the infra-orbital nerves.

On Inspection Intra-orally.—There is gagging of the occlusion in the molar area and retroposition of the upper incisors in relation to the lower teeth. The upper midline may be deviated to one side and the entire occlusal plane may be dropped down, forcing the mandible open. If this has happened the mandible is widely open and the patient is complaining that he 'cannot open the mouth' (*Figs.* 18, 19).

If the middle third of the facial skeleton has been pushed back very far, the soft palate will be resting on the dorsum of the tongue and the oral airway may be occluded.

There is often marked ecchymosis in the buccal sulcus over the zygomatic buttress.

The maxillae may be split apart up the midline and associated alveolar fractures or injuries to one or more teeth may be present.

On Palpation.—The tooth-bearing segment is found to be freely mobile, especially if there is an associated Le Fort I type fracture present. It is usually possible to reposition it by gentle manipulation without anaesthesia. If the tooth-bearing fragment has dropped it is often possible to raise it as much as 2 in. or 5 cm.—again without anaesthetic.

Palpation in the zygomatic buttress area often reveals crepitus and tapping of the teeth elicits the 'cracked cup' sound.

Summary of Symptoms.—
1. Gross swelling of face.
2. Two black eyes.
3. Deformity of nose.
4. Lengthening of face.
5. Face appears flat.
6. Face feels loose.
7. Double vision.
8. Numbness of cheeks.
9. Gagging of back teeth.
10. Front teeth not meeting.

Summary of Physical Signs.—
1. Gross oedema of soft tissues over middle third of facial skeleton.
2. Bilateral circumorbital ecchymosis.
3. Bilateral subconjunctival ecchymosis of outer and possibly inner halves of the eye.
4. Limitation of ocular movements.
5. Diplopia.
6. Possibly enophthalmos.
7. Anaesthesia of cheeks.
8. Obvious displacement of nasal structures.
9. Flattening of face.
10. Displacement of zygomatic bones.
11. Lengthening of face.
12. Mobility of zygomatic bones.
13. Mobility of facial skeleton.
14. Epistaxis.
15. Possibly cerebrospinal fluid rhinorrhoea.
16. Retroposition of upper incisors.
17. Gagging of occlusion in molar area.
18. Anterior open bite.
19. Occlusion of oral airway by soft palate being forced down on dorsum of tongue.

20. Mandible wide open and patient incapable of separating lower and upper teeth, the upper jaw having fallen.

UNILATERAL LE FORT I, II, AND III TYPE FRACTURES.—It is possible for a unilateral fracture of the middle third of the facial skeleton to occur, and it may be of the Le Fort I, II, or III variety.

The physical signs are similar to those already described, but they are, of course, only present on one side.

Immobilization by extra-oral or internal skeletal fixation is facilitated by the presence of intact skeletal tissue on the unaffected side.

CHAPTER VII

CEREBROSPINAL FLUID RHINORRHOEA

THE possibility of a cerebrospinal fluid rhinorrhoea should be considered in Le Fort II and III type fractures and in severe naso-ethmoidal damage. In such injuries the cribriform plate of the ethmoid is shattered and if there is an associated dural tear cerebrospinal fluid will escape down the nostril. The early recognition of this condition is difficult in the recently injured subject owing to the presence of blood-clots in the nares. In the early stage the cerebrospinal fluid is masked by epistaxis, and when the blood clots it may act as a temporary plug. Later, when the clot becomes organized, there may be a discharge of clear serum which can be mistaken for cerebrospinal fluid. If the patient has been suffering from acute coryza before the injury, or develops the condition shortly afterwards, this nasal discharge, too, may cause confusion.

However, any clear watery fluid which is seen to drip from the nostril should be considered to be a cerebrospinal fluid leak and the appropriate tests should be carried out. Sometimes the cerebrospinal fluid escapes down the throat and, under these circumstances, the patient complains of a salty taste.

Determination of the protein content of the escaping fluid is useful in differentiating between cerebrospinal fluid and the serum from the blood-clot, because cerebrospinal fluid contains little protein. Nasal secretions from acute coryza contain mucin but no sugar, while the reverse is true in the case of cerebrospinal fluid.

Cerebrospinal fluid rhinorrhoea may also occur as a result of a fracture through the base of the sphenoid communicating with the sphenoidal sinus and through a crack in the roof of this structure with the cisterna chiasmatica. It is usually necessary for a neurosurgeon to perform a fascia lata repair in order to correct such a leak.

Incidence of Cerebrospinal Fluid Rhinorrhoea.—Lewin and Cairns (1951) showed that 84 out of 308 head injuries, or 27·3 per cent, had cerebrospinal fluid rhinorrhoea.

Lewin, in a further series, showed 18 out of 72, or 25 per cent.

Dawson and Fordyce (1953), in their review of 190 cases of middle third injuries, had 45, or 24 per cent, with cerebrospinal fluid rhinorrhoea.

Rowe and Killey (1968) had 60 cases with 14, or 23·3 per cent, with cerebrospinal fluid rhinorrhoea.

The onset of this condition may be delayed, but is usually present within 48 hours. Lewin reports its onset in occasional cases some months after injury.

The duration of the condition again varies according to these authorities, but usually lasts about a week. Dawson and Fordyce give an average of 9 days; Rowe and Killey, 5 to 7 days. Lewin, dealing with cases which are primarily head injuries, gives an average of 7 days for the majority of cases, but occasionally the duration may be protracted, even to the extent of months.

In the absence of intracranial complications, such as an intracranial haemorrhage, one of the most important factors in arresting a cerebrospinal fluid leak is the repositioning and immobilization of the facial fractures. Fixation is especially valuable as it prevents the pumping action of a mobile middle-third fracture which, in the cribriform plate area, may pump infection up through the torn dura and produce meningitis. This pumping action will also occur if mandibular/maxillary fixation is carried out without first immobilizing the mobile upper jaw.

There is much divergence of opinion as to whether a dural repair should be carried out. Calvert (1942) considered that all cases should have a dural repair, but this opinion was given in the pre-antibiotic era. Meredith (1951) considered it necessary when the cerebrospinal fluid leak had persisted for 10 days or more. Dandy (1945) considered that the condition should not be allowed to persist for more than 10 days.

O'Connell (1968) considers that a cerebrospinal fluid leak which persists for more than two weeks probably requires exploration and closure of the fistula. With leaks of shorter duration he believes that spontaneous healing of the torn meninges will provide an effective barrier against infection.

Fistulae occur most commonly in the frontal sinus area and are least common in the sphenoid. Neurosurgeons tend to be more conservative in their treatment of fistulae which are sited toward the sphenoid area, for surgical access to this region is difficult.

The problem is related, of course, to the possibility of meningitis occurring as a late complication. Lewin shows that there is a 25 per cent risk of meningitis developing in cases where a cerebrospinal fluid rhinorrhoea has ceased spontaneously and where no dural repair has been carried out.

Statistics from the maxillo-facial units do not confirm such a high figure for late meningitis, but it is reasonable to suppose that many cases which develop such a complication are not referred back to the units which treated the middle-third fractures and so are lost to their statistics. Many of the cases of meningitis occur years after the cerebrospinal fluid leak, and in the circumstances it might be appropriate to secure a neurosurgical opinion in the case of all patients who have had a cerebrospinal fluid rhinorrhoea. A long-term follow-up is also necessary in these cases, and the patient's own medical practitioner should be informed of the possibility of such a late complication.

Prophylactic Measures.—Penicillin does not cross the blood meningeal barrier in therapeutically effective concentration and as a prophylactic measure all patients suffering from injuries which could produce a cerebrospinal fluid leak should have sulphadiazine by mouth or, if unconscious, by injection. The chemotherapy should be continued until 48 hours after any cerebrospinal fluid leak has ceased or until the patient is found to have no such complication. The chemotherapy is given in conjunction with any antibiotic therapy which may be considered advisable in treating associated injuries.

CHAPTER VIII

RADIOLOGY FOR FRACTURES OF THE MIDDLE THIRD OF THE FACIAL SKELETON

A CAREFUL clinical examination of the injury combined with an intimate knowledge of the surgical anatomy of the area enables the clinician to diagnose the nature of the fractures with a high degree of accuracy. It is, therefore, unnecessary to subject an ill patient to a protracted radiological examination, but when the patient's general condition permits, good-quality radiographs should be obtained with minimum discomfort and inconvenience to the patient. A thorough radiological examination should never be omitted, as there are certain injuries, such as a fractured cervical spine or a depressed fracture of the vault of the skull, which cannot be readily detected on clinical examination alone and may have some considerable influence on the subsequent course of treatment.

When the patient is considered to be fit for X-ray examination, the radiography should be carried out rapidly and efficiently by a radiographer experienced in this work, and care should be taken to see that the patient is kept warm and that the examination is planned so that minimum disturbance of the patient is necessary.

The use of a skull unit, such as a Schönander or Barazzetti, is valuable as the patient can be radiographed in a sitting position and does not have to lie with the fractured face against the X-ray couch.

The radiographs required are:—

1. Occipito-mental, 15°, 30°, and 45°.
2. Submento-vertical.
3. True lateral.
4. Occlusal view of maxillae.
5. Intra-orals.
6. Cranial views, postero-anterior and lateral.

Isolated fractures of the orbital floor cannot be demonstrated with accuracy on the routine occipito-mental radiographs and Milauskas (1969) recommends the use of the 30° postero-anterior and the 20°/35° oblique view to demonstrate these injuries. Regular linear tomography is of limited value in the diagnosis of orbital floor fractures due to the presence of streaking parasite shadows which make the tomograms difficult to interpret. Orbital floor fractures are best demonstrated by polytomography (hypocycloid tomography).

Milauskas (1969) considers that orbitograms have a diagnostic accuracy of approximately 95% as confirmed by surgical exploration. In this technique an injection of hypaque is made along the orbital floor in the extraconal space. If a fracture is present the contrast material flows down into the maxillary sinus.

Good stereoscopic radiographs are difficult to obtain during the immediate post-traumatic period but they are occasionally most helpful in demonstrating the exact nature of the displacements.

Chapter IX

OUTLINE OF DEFINITIVE TREATMENT OF FRACTURES OF THE MIDDLE THIRD OF THE FACIAL SKELETON

THE definitive treatment of fractures of the middle third of the facial skeleton must, of necessity, vary according to the type of fracture. Basically, it does not differ from the treatment of fractures elsewhere in the body, and consists of the reduction of the fracture and immobilization of the fragments until bony union has occurred. There has, in the past, been some controversy as to whether bony union does, in fact, occur in fractures of the middle third, or whether such injuries result in a fibrous union.

As has already been pointed out in the section on surgical anatomy, the middle third is made up of a number of slender bony struts running upwards in the general direction of the base of the skull. After repositioning middle-third injuries, some of these bony struts will be in contact and some will be separated. Where the bone is in contact with bone, there will be bony union, but if in some areas the bones are separated by an excessive distance, there may be a fibrous union. The greater part of the union will, however, be bony.

DENTO-ALVEOLAR FRACTURES

Fractured Teeth without Exposure of the Pulp.—These are pulp tested and X-rayed. Death of the pulp occurs as a late complication in a number of these teeth, and they should be reviewed at intervals so that if the pulp dies, root filling is performed. Suitable conservative treatment is carried out to restore the appearance.

Fractured Teeth with Exposure of the Pulp.—The exposed pulp should be touched with phenol on a small pledget of cotton-wool to relieve the patient of any acute pain, and then a decision has to be made as to whether to root fill the tooth and carry out restorative treatment or to extract the tooth. Comminuted teeth and teeth fractured beneath the gum must be extracted.

Subluxated Teeth.—Slightly subluxated teeth, provided they are in a good position, should be left alone if firm or splinted if they are mobile. They often become firm and retain their vitality, especially in young patients. Follow-up pulp testing and X-ray examinations should be carried out. If the tooth is severely subluxated, death of the pulp will inevitably result if it is pushed back into its correct position. If such a tooth is replaced and splinted, root filling is carried out, if and when the tooth becomes firm.

If the tooth is avulsed or subluxated to the extent that it can be picked out of its socket with the fingers, it can be root filled from the root end, after which the apex is cut off and the tooth replanted and splinted in position. A tooth so treated usually becomes firm but resorption of the root eventually leads to its loss. However, a tooth may be preserved for months and sometimes even years by these means and, occasionally, such treatment is worth while.

Fractures of the Alveolus.—

Fractures of the Maxillary Tuberosity: If the tuberosity is completely detached from the periosteum it should be carefully dissected out and the resulting soft-tissue defect carefully sutured to prevent any residual opening into the maxillary sinus.

If the tuberosity with or without associated teeth appears to be attached to the periosteum, the tuberosity can be left alone with or without splinting. Splinting of the tooth attached to the fragment and immobilizing it to other standing teeth in the maxilla for one month usually results in union, but if the tooth in the tuberosity fragment requires extraction it should

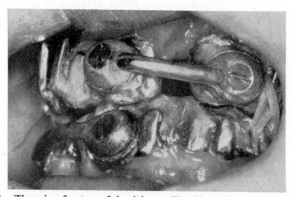

Fig. 20.—There is a fracture of the right maxilla which is immobilized to the intact left side by a silver/copper alloy cap splint and connecting bar. A fracture in the lower jaw has also been treated with splints and a connecting bar.

be removed surgically by drilling away the surrounding bone after the tuberosity is firm. If the tooth is painful, this surgical extraction must be carried out earlier, but the chance of saving the tuberosity in such circumstances is greatly reduced.

Fractures of the alveolar floor of the maxillary sinus are treated in the same way, depending upon whether the alveolar fragment, together with any associated teeth, is completely detached from the periosteum.

If the alveolus and floor of the antrum are inadvertently removed, as during the extraction of teeth, a very careful soft-tissue repair of the defect must be carried out immediately, if necessary by advancing a buccal flap. The patient should be given nasal inhalations of Tinct. Benzoin Co., and nasal drops of ephedrine ½–1 per cent along with an antibiotic for 7 days to ensure antral drainage during healing, and to prevent breakdown and development of an oro-antral fistula.

Sometimes there is an extensive fracture of the alveolus with several teeth attached. This can be treated by splinting the teeth and anchoring the splint to teeth elsewhere in the upper jaw. (*Fig.* 20.) In the incisor area these cap splints can be made of acrylic, which is shaded and contoured to resemble the incisor teeth. Such splints are fixed to the teeth with crown-and-bridge cement and are aesthetically acceptable to the patient.

As an immediate measure, loose teeth can be splinted by using an arch bar fitted to the upper teeth and secured to the loose tooth by 0·35-mm. soft stainless-steel wire. To prevent the loose tooth being avulsed when the wire securing it to the arch bar is tightened, a small wire attachment should be soldered to the arch bar and extended over the incisal tip of the loose tooth, so holding it into the socket.

Comminuted fractures of the alveolus in the incisor area, with or without comminution of associated teeth, usually necessitate the removal of the portions of teeth and alveolus and careful soft-tissue repair of the resulting alveolar defect. The operator should preserve any portions of alveolus which appear to have a chance of survival. Lacerated wounds in the lip should be carefully explored, and any fragments of teeth removed; then the edges of the wound are trimmed and closure carried out.

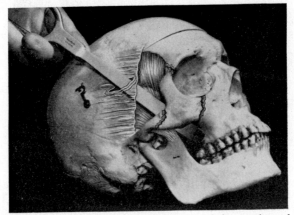

Fig. 21.—Diagram to show Bristow's elevator being used to elevate a fractured zygomatic bone. The instrument is passed through an incision in the temporalis fascia and down on to the temporalis muscle beneath the zygomatic bone.

ZYGOMATIC COMPLEX FRACTURES

Fractures of the zygomatic complex require reduction for the following reasons:—

1. If the patient has diplopia.
2. When there is limitation of mandibular movements.
3. In order to restore the normal skeletal protection for the globe of the eye.
4. The last, and least important, reason for operating upon these fractures is the cosmetic result.

Zygomatic complex fractures with minimal displacement which are not causing symptoms do not require treatment. In a series of 336 fractures of the zygomatic complex (Rowe and Killey, 1968), 66 or 19·64 per cent required no surgical treatment. Sometimes a more severely displaced zygomatic bone is left if the patient is elderly and a poor operative risk.

Cases with diplopia always require operation, but old zygomatic bone or arch fractures which have become united and are causing limitation of mandibular movements can be treated by performing a coronoidectomy.

Reduction.—Reduction of a recent fracture is carried out from the Gillies approach (Gillies, Kilner, and Stone, 1927), The surgical anatomy underlying this operation depends upon the fact that, whereas the temporal fascia is attached along the superior surface of the zygomatic arch, the

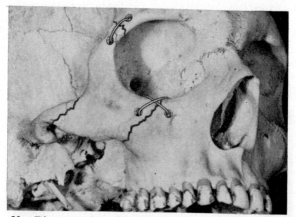

Fig. 22.—Diagram of transosseous wiring at zygomatico-frontal and zygomatico-maxillary fracture lines. Transosseous wiring is commonly employed at these sites. The twisted end of wire is inserted into one of the holes.

temporalis muscle passes beneath the arch to be attached to the coronoid process and down the ramus as far as the retromolar fossa. Therefore, if an incision is made in the hairline in the temporal region and the temporal fascia is incised, it is possible to pass an instrument down on to the temporalis muscle beneath the zygomatic arch. The zygomatic bone or its arch can then be elevated into its correct position.

An incision about 2 cm. long is made between the bifurcation of the two branches of the superficial temporal vein and the temporalis fascia is exposed and then incised. A Bristow's elevator is passed down beneath the zygomatic bone which is then gently lifted back into position (*Fig.* 21).

In the recent fracture, the fragment is stable after reduction as the fractured ends of the zygomatic bone and maxilla interdigitate.

The temporal fascia is sutured with catgut and the skin with silk.

Some operators prefer to elevate the zygomatic bone from an intra-oral approach through an incision in the buccal sulcus. Others make an external incision and pass a hook under the bone, but, in practice, the Gillies approach will be found simple to perform and gives good control over the zygomatic bone during reduction—it is the method of choice.

Following reduction, the bone may be stable or additional fixation is required. Instability of the fragment commonly occurs when there has been delay in treatment: the fractured ends of the bone tend to become rounded off by osteoclastic activity and after the zygomatic bone has been elevated into place it falls back into its original position.

Control of the unstable zygomatic bone fracture may be achieved by:—

1. *Transosseous Wiring at the Zygomatico-frontal Fracture Line:* The zygomatico-frontal fracture line is exposed by blunt dissection through a small incision in one of the skin wrinkles at the corner of the eye. Small holes are drilled in the zygomatic process of the frontal bone and the frontal process of the zygomatic bone, and after the fracture has been reduced, the zygomatic bone is fixed in position by a piece of 0·5-mm. soft stainless-steel wire which is passed through the two holes and tied. Accurate reduction and immobilization can be achieved by this method.

The fracture area can also be approached through a semilunar incision with its convex surface upwards which is made through the eyebrow. The scar will be invisible when the hair grows over the area.

2. *Transosseous Wiring at the Zygomatico-maxillary Fracture Line:* An approach to the zygomatico-maxillary fracture line is made through a semilunar incision about $\frac{1}{2}$ in. or 1·25 cm. long, made through the skin just beneath the lower orbital rim. Again holes are drilled in the adjacent fragments, the fracture is reduced, and fixation is achieved by wiring (*Fig.* 22).

3. *A Combination of Zygomatico-frontal and Zygomatico-maxillary Wiring* may be used.

4. *Fixation with a Pack in the Maxillary Sinus:* An approach is made to the maxillary sinus through an incision in the buccal sulcus. On exposing the bone a hole into the maxillary sinus is usually seen to be present as a result of the fracture, otherwise a window into the sinus is made through the canine fossa. The opening into the maxillary sinus is enlarged and the blood-clot and fragments of bone within it are evacuated. The zygomatic bone is repositioned from this intra-oral approach, or if a Gillies approach has already been made, the bone can be elevated with a Bristow's elevator. The operator gently repositions any fragments of the orbital floor with his finger, then the antrum is packed with $\frac{1}{2}$-in. or 1·25-cm. ribbon gauze soaked in 1–1000 acriflavine or Whitehead's varnish in order to hold the zygomatic bone in position. The end of the pack is left protruding from the incision in the buccal sulcus and is sutured to the edge of the wound. An acriflavine pack tends to become infected after about a couple of weeks but it is an easy pack to remove when treatment is completed. The Whitehead's varnish pack will remain uninfected for several weeks. It is very stable, and, contrary to general belief, no difficulty will be experienced in removing it at the completion of treatment. Maxillary sinus packs are normally left in place for about three weeks, and then removed through the original incision in the buccal sulcus. The wound in the sulcus closes without the necessity of further surgery. Great care must be taken in packing the antrum not to displace any bony spicules of the orbital floor against the optic nerve and ophthalmic artery. The optic nerve is a relatively strong structure, but a spicule of bone touching the ophthalmic artery may cause spasm of the vessel, and subsequent loss of vision due to damage to the retina.

For this reason the pack should be directed chiefly to the outer aspect of the antrum beneath the zygomatic bone, and it should not be packed too tightly on the medial aspect of the antrum beneath the optic nerve and ophthalmic artery.

For the same reason, when there is an associated Le Fort II or III type fracture, this should be reduced and immobilized before packing the antrum in order to provide fixation for an unstable fractured zygomatic bone. If the antrum is packed and then the middle third of the face is manipulated, the antral pack will be forced against the orbital floor and damage to the orbital contents may lead to loss of vision.

Antral packing is only effective if the bony fragments of the orbital floor remain attached to the periosteum and it is obviously useless to pack the maxillary sinus if the bony fragments are lost and there is a hole in the floor of the orbit. In such cases a bone-graft or Teflon implant to the orbital floor is indicated.

Balloons or a Foley catheter in the antrum have been used instead of a pack, but they have the disadvantage that they expand uniformly in all directions and pressure cannot be exerted in the correct sites with any degree of accuracy. The balloon devices are inserted through an intra-nasal antrostomy and are filled with a radio-opaque fluid.

5. *Pin Fixation from the Zygomatic Bone to a Plaster-of-Paris Headcap:* In this technique, two thin bone pins are inserted into the zygomatic bone. The fracture is reduced and then the two pins are connected to a plaster-of-Paris headcap by connecting rods and universal joints.

This technique is especially useful in the zygomatic bone which is excessively mobile following reduction and it is the only possible method of fixation following surgical refracture of a badly displaced zygomatic bone which has healed.

Two pins are used in order to prevent rotation of the zygomatic bone which would occur if only one pin was used. Some operators advocate the use of one 'wood' screw type pin for this purpose.

Pin fixation of the zygomatic bone can also be effected by fitting a cap splint to the upper teeth and having a rod extension from this splint connected to the pins in the zygomatic bone.

6. If the zygomatic bone is comminuted, direct wiring of the fragments may be carried out through an appropriate incision.

In an analysis of 336 zygomatic bone fractures (Rowe and Killey, 1968) 235 were treated by simple elevation, 18 required transosseous wiring, 8 had pin fixation to a plaster-of-Paris headcap, and the maxillary sinus was packed in 9 cases; 66 cases required no active surgical treatment.

Necessity for Fixation of the Mandible in Zygomatic Fractures.—It is unnecessary to immobilize the mandible by mandibular-maxillary fixation in a zygomatic complex fracture, though some authorities advocate such a measure to counter the action of the masseter muscle, but the temporalis fascia attached along the superior surface of the zygomatic arch usually prevents the masseter from pulling the fragments down. If, for some reason, the temporalis fascia was stripped from the arch, then mandibular-maxillary fixation would be advisable.

Fractures of the Zygomatic Arch.—If the zygomatic arch alone is fractured, the fragments should be reduced via a Gillies approach. Fixation is unnecessary as the temporalis fascia attached along the superior aspect of the arch will effectively immobilize the fragments.

FRACTURES OF THE ORBITAL FLOOR.—Fractures of the orbital floor may occur in association with fractures of the zygomatic complex or in isolated fractures of the orbit (Converse, 1957), when only the orbital floor is fractured.

Fractures of the orbital floor lead to herniation of the periorbital fat into the maxillary sinus which results in enophthalmos. The inferior oblique and inferior rectus muscles may become incarcerated in the fracture line and diplopia results.

Treatment.—According to Rowe (1973) once the diagnosis of fracture of the orbital floor has been established, surgical intervention is indicated in all but the most minor degrees of displacement. Goldberg (1969) considers that exploration is indicated only if there is significant enophthalmos, limitation of movement or marked incarceration of orbital tissue as demonstrated radiographically.

Certainly surgery in the form of bone or allelograft to the orbital floor has become increasingly popular in recent times but it is difficult to assess the necessity or the effect of many of the results. In most cases of zygomatic bone fracture there is an associated fracture of the orbital floor. For many years these fractures have been treated by simple reposition of the zygomatic bone without special attention to the orbital floor, except in some gross cases where the maxillary sinus was packed. Analysis of the results achieved has shown few cases of residual diplopia and most of these have been successfully corrected by ophthalmic surgery to the orbital muscles concerned. Van Herk and Hovinga (1973) have analysed 115 cases of isolated fracture of the orbital floor which recovered with no orbital complications and they state that implants to the orbital floor are unnecessary in the treatment of recent fractures. Grafting of the orbital floor is by no means free from severe complications, such as retrobulbar haemorrhage. Goldberg (1969) lists the following complications of this operation at the time of surgery: (1) Inability to extricate all incarcerated tissue, (2) Avulsion of inferior rectus or inferior oblique, (3) Mistaken identification of infra-orbital nerve, (4) Excessive pressure on globe. The post-operative complications may be: (5) Bacterial contamination, (6) Persistent limitation in vertical gaze, (7) Persistent exophthalmos, (8) Enophthalmos, (9) Extrusion of alloplastic sheet, (10) Lower lid extropion, (11) Post-operative lid oedema, (12) Dacrocystitis.

Hotte (1970) has stated that when an implant is placed on the orbital floor there is no certainty that it will prevent enophthalmos. Lyle (1963) has pointed out that, in a comprehensive survey, from the standpoint of the ophthalmic surgeon diplopia may persist even though restoration of the ocular level and elimination of fibrous adhesions between the globe and the orbital floor have been successfully accomplished.

Finally, it is difficult to assess a successful result following immediate grafting to the orbital floor and be certain that a similar satisfactory outcome would not have occurred without surgery. In view of the difficulty in deciding which cases require active surgical intervention all orbital floor fractures should be treated both pre- and post-operatively in conjunction with a consultant ophthalmic surgeon.

When there is doubt concerning the interpretation of the various clinical and radiological investigations Rowe (1973) suggests performing a

Caldwell-Luc operation to ascertain the exact extent of the injury by direct inspection of the orbital floor. If the depressed fragments are attached to the periosteum they can be repositioned by gentle digital manipulations, and if there is no actual bone loss the sinus is evacuated of its blood-clot and packed with 1-cm. ribbon gauze soaked in Whitehead's varnish. The end of the pack is left protruding from the wound in the buccal sulcus and can be withdrawn in three weeks, after which the Caldwell-Luc incision will heal spontaneously. It is important not to pack into the postero-medial superior aspect of the maxillary sinus which lies beneath the optic nerve.

If inspection of the orbital floor confirms that there is actual bone loss a graft to the orbital floor is indicated. An incision is made in a natural skin crease immediately below the lid margin. The incision should not be extended too far laterally as it may interfere with lymphatic drainage. The skin is dissected off the orbicularis oculi muscle which is then split tangentially at a slightly lower level than the original incision. The periosteum is incised and the orbital contents are supported with a blunt retractor while the orbital tissues are eased upwards through the defect in the orbital floor. The bony gap is then covered with a 0·5–1 mm. thick sheet of Silastic or Teflon cut to a triangular shape and sufficiently large to be supported at its periphery on sound bone. The periosteum is then sutured to prevent extrusion of the graft and the skin incision is closed. Alternatively, autogenous bone may be used for this purpose.

Nasal Complex Fractures

Reduction.—Nasal complex fractures may be reduced under local analgesia, but general anaesthesia with a peroral endotracheal tube and adequate throat pack is desirable because haemorrhage may be profuse.

Walsham's and Asche's forceps are used for manipulating the fragments. The unpadded blade of the Walsham's forceps is passed up the nostril

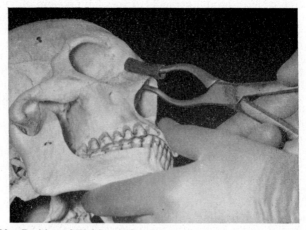

Fig. 23.—Position of Walsham's forceps when reducing fractures of the nasal complex.

and the nasal bone and associated fragment of the frontal process of the maxilla are secured between it and the padded blade externally (*Fig.* 23). The fragments are manipulated into their correct position and then the manœuvre is repeated on the opposite side.

Next, the vomer and the perpendicular plate of the ethmoid are 'ironed out' with the Asche's septal forceps, using one blade each side of the septum and then, if possible, the septal cartilage is grasped and brought forwards and repositioned in its groove in the vomer. Next, the finger and thumb of one hand are used to compress the lacrimal bones and medial walls of the orbit on each side to achieve a narrow bridge to the nose.

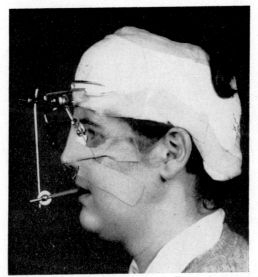

Fig. 24.—Nasal plaster held in position with Elastoplast strapping. Note that the nasal splint must not be connected to the plaster-of-Paris headcap.

Finally, an instrument should be passed down each of the nares to ensure that they are clear and that the patient has a patent nasal airway.

If the nasal complex region is severely comminuted, it is often sufficient to mould the nose into shape between the thumb and forefinger or by applying a thumb along each side of the nose and squeezing. Such fractures tend to be less stable after reduction.

Fixation.—Sometimes when the fracture is not very severe it is unnecessary to splint the nose following the reduction. Usually, however, some sort of splint fixation is advisable.

The most commonly used splint is a plaster-of-Paris splint consisting of eight layers of plaster-of-Paris bandage cut so as to produce a strip of plaster across the bridge and covering either side of the nose, with an extension up to and along the forehead.

The plaster-of-Paris bandage splint is moulded into place while wet and held while it sets, and then it is fixed into position with strips of

Elastoplast across the forehead and down each side of the nose (*Fig.* 24). It is important never to connect such a nasal plaster to a plaster-of-Paris headcap for, if the headcap rides down on the forehead a little, it produces a depressed bridge of the nose because the subsidence is transmitted to the nasal splint.

When the oedema over the nasal region has subsided in about a week, it is prudent to apply a fresh, accurately fitting nasal plaster. The nasal plaster should be left in situ for about three weeks only.

If the nasal fracture is too mobile to be efficiently splinted with plaster-of-Paris, a lead plate splint either side of the nose is used. Two lead plates, each with an upper and lower hole through the centre, are fitted

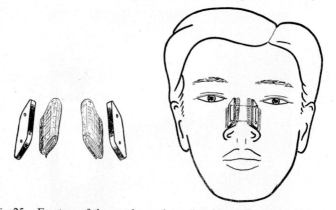

Fig. 25.—Fracture of the nasal complex splinted between two lead plates which are held in position by a mattress suture of stainless-steel or tantalum wire. Pads of cotton-wool are placed beneath the metal plates so that the underlying skin is not excoriated.

either side of the nose with a cotton-wool roll beneath the plates to prevent them chafing the skin. They are held in position by a mattress suture of tantalum or 0·35-mm. soft stainless-steel wire which is passed through the holes in the lead plates, the wires transfixing the tissues and passing beneath the nasal bones. (*Fig.* 25.)

This splint is left in situ for about three weeks. Occasionally, if the nasal complex region is particularly flat, it is necessary to attach this nasal splint by wire to an anterior connecting rod from a plaster-of-Paris headcap to hold the nose forward. Elastic traction may be used to achieve this result when there has been a delay in treating such a case.

LE FORT I, II, AND III TYPE FRACTURES

1. LE FORT I, GUÉRIN, OR LOW-LEVEL FRACTURES.—

Reduction.—Reduction of these fractures is carried out by grasping the tooth-bearing portion of the upper jaw and manipulating it into its correct position. If there are teeth present, this will, of course, be when normal occlusion is restored. If the fragment is very loose, this manœuvre can occasionally be carried out with finger pressure alone. Usually, however, it is necessary to manipulate the fragment by gripping it between the blades of two pairs of Walsham's forceps or Rowe's disimpaction forceps. The unpadded blade is passed up the nostril, and the padded blade enters the mouth and grips the palate. Standing behind the patient, the operator grips the handles of the two pairs of forceps and manipulates the fragments into place.

If the fragment is firmly impacted, it may be necessary to expose the fracture line through an incision in the buccal sulcus and mobilize it with an osteotome before applying the forceps.

2. LE FORT II, PYRAMIDAL, OR SUB-ZYGOMATIC FRACTURES.—
Reduction.—The tooth-bearing portion of the upper jaw is grasped between two pairs of Walsham's forceps or Rowe's disimpaction forceps (*Fig.* 26), one unpadded blade of each forcep being inserted in the nostril and the other padded blade passing into the mouth to grip the palate. If the section of bone is more or less in one main piece, it should be gently

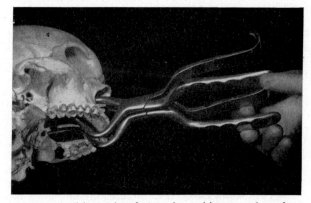

Fig. 26.—Rowe's disimpaction forceps in position to reduce the tooth-bearing portion of the upper jaw.

rocked free and manipulated upwards and forwards up the inclined plane formed by the frontal bone and body of the sphenoid. Usually, however, there is an associated low-level or Le Fort I type fracture, and this segment moves independently of the main fragment. The tooth-bearing fragment is brought upwards and forwards until the occlusion is judged to be normal. At this stage, the space on opening between the upper and lower incisor teeth is about the width of three of the operator's fingers.

When the tooth-bearing portion is adequately reduced, this fragment is immobilized and then the associated naso-ethmoidal section is reduced and fixed.

3. LE FORT III, HIGH-LEVEL, OR SUPRA-ZYGOMATIC TYPE FRACTURES.—
Reduction.—These severe injuries usually comprise Le Fort I, II, and III type fractures associated with bilateral zygomatic complex and nasal complex fractures.

Disimpaction should be carried out in the following order:—

a. First the zygomatic bones are elevated for it is impossible to disimpact the central Le Fort II portion with the zygomatic bones depressed.

Sometimes this elevation of the zygomatic bone can be effected from the buccal sulcus, or it may be necessary to carry out its elevation via the Gillies approach.

b. Next, the tooth-bearing portion of the upper jaw is reduced by grasping it between two pairs of Walsham's or Rowe's disimpaction forceps, one blade up the nostril and one into the palate, and manipulating it upwards and forwards until the normal occlusion and adequate mandibular opening is achieved. When the tooth-bearing portion is in a satisfactory position, fixation is carried out.

c. The naso-ethmoidal section is then repositioned and finally the zygomatic complex and the nasal complex sections are immobilized.

If it is necessary to pack a maxillary sinus, this is carried out after all other treatment is completed, and no further manipulation of the facial skeleton should be carried out with an antral pack in position. Manipulation of the facial skeleton at this stage may cause severe damage to the eye for the antral pack is pushed through the fractured orbital floor.

IMMOBILIZATION OF LE FORT I, II, AND III TYPE FRACTURES

General Considerations.—The fixation of a mobile fracture of the middle third of the facial skeleton presents a difficult problem as there is no suitable adjacent structure to which it can be immobilized.

A number of ingenious methods of fixation have been evolved to overcome this difficulty. These can be divided into two main groups: (1) *Extra-oral immobilization*, and (2) *Immobilization within the tissues*.

1. *Extra-oral Immobilization:* This is achieved in two ways:—

a. *Suspension:* The mobile portion of the upper jaw may be suspended from a plaster-of-Paris headcap by an arrangement of connecting bars and splints. If the upper jaw is connected to the headcap, the method is known as 'cranio-maxillary fixation', and if the lower jaw is connected to the headcap, so sandwiching the fractured middle third between the mandible and the base of the skull, the immobilization is called 'craniomandibular fixation' (*Figs.* 27–29).

b. *Indirect skeletal fixation:* This is achieved by inserting external pins into the mandible and connecting them by rods and universal joints to pins in the zygomatic bones or the frontal bone. This form of treatment is effective provided the pins do not become loosened.

A similar fixation can be achieved by transfixing the mandible with a Kirschner wire or Steinmann pin, and connecting it by rods and universal joints to the same wire or pin transfixing the zygomatic bones.

2. *Immobilization within the Tissues:* This is achieved by direct fixation, suspension, and support.

a. *Direct fixation:* Fixation is achieved either by transosseous wiring at the zygomatico-frontal, zygomatico-maxillary, zygomatic, and midline of palate fracture sites, or by transfixation with a Kirschner wire through both zygomas and the maxillae or by two Kirschner wires driven from each zygomatic bone into the nasal septum.

b. *The suspension techniques* involve connecting the lower jaw by wires to areas of the facial skeleton above the fracture line, so sandwiching the fractured portion between the mandible and that part of the facial skeleton which is not involved in the fracture.

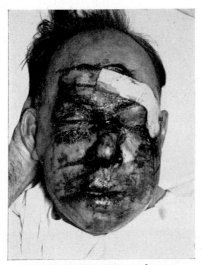

Fig. 27.—Le Fort III type fracture.

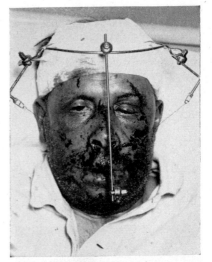

Fig. 28.—Fixation employed in treatment of fracture shown in Fig. 27.

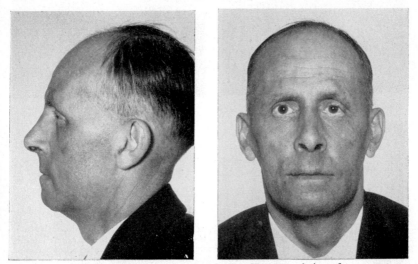

Fig. 29.—Profile and full face of patient in Fig. 27 at completion of treatment.

c. *Support* is achieved by packing the maxillary sinus or by the use of balloons in the antrum.

These forms of immobilization may be classified as follows:—

1. *Extra-oral Immobilization:*
a. *Suspension from a plaster-of-Paris headcap:*
  i. Cranio-maxillary.

  ii. Cranio-mandibular.
 b. Indirect skeletal fixation:
  i. Zygomatico-mandibular.
  ii. Fronto-mandibular.
 2. *Immobilization within the Tissues:*
 a. Direct fixation by:
  i. Transosseous wiring at fracture sites:
    This may be:—
     α. Zygomatico-frontal.
     β. Zygomatico-maxillary.
     γ. Comminuted zygomatic bone.
     δ. Midline of palate.
  ii. Transfixation with Kirschner wire:
     α. Zygomatico-maxillary.
     β. Zygomatico-septal.

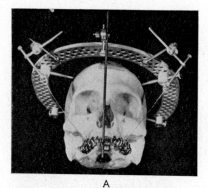

A

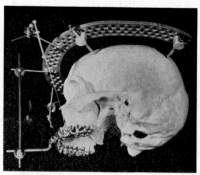

B

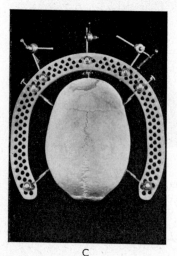

C

Fig. 30.—The Royal Berkshire Hospital halo frame. A, Full face; B, Tilted lateral; and C, View from above to show the pins placed co-axially and mounted in similar numbered holes in the frame.

b. *Suspension by wires:*
   i. Circumzygomatic.
  ii. Zygomatico-mandibular.
 iii. Inferior orbital border-mandibular.
  iv. Fronto-mandibular.
   v. Pyriform fossa-mandibular.
  vi. Nasal septum.
c. *Support:*
   i. Antral packs.
  ii. Antral balloons.

NOTES ON THE VARIOUS METHODS OF FIXATION.—
Extra-oral Immobilization.—
   1. *Suspension from a Plaster-of-Paris Headcap:* No plaster-of-Paris headcap is absolutely stable, but in practice an efficiently applied headcap provides an adequate fixed point to which the upper jaw can be immobilized.

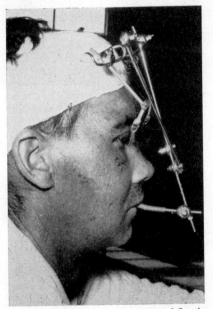

Fig. 31.—Le Fort III type fracture treated by external fixation with a plaster-of-Paris headcap, transbuccal cheek wires, and an anterior connecting rod to a projecting bar from an upper cap splint.

Absolute stability can be achieved by using the 'halo' type head frame which is secured directly to the skull by screw pins which perforate the scalp to contact the outer cortical plate. This type of apparatus was devised by Crawford (1943) and was modified by Perry and Nickel (1959) and Thompson (1962) for use in the treatment of cervical spine injuries. Panuska and Dedolph (1965) recommended its use in the treatment of facial fractures. The Crewe (1966) type of head frame encircles the head and is attached to the skull by four pins. It has the disadvantage that it projects backwards from the occiput and prevents the patient from lying comfortably with the back of the head on a pillow. This problem is

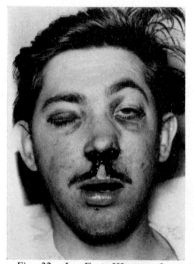

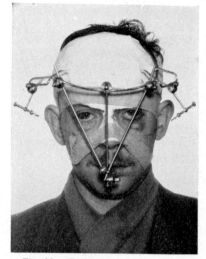

Fig. 32.—Le Fort III type fracture. Note lengthening of face and deviation of nasal complex to the left. There has been some fall in the level of the left eye with the upper lid following it down, producing the physical sign of ' hooding '.

Fig. 33.—Fracture shown in Fig. 32, showing fixation.

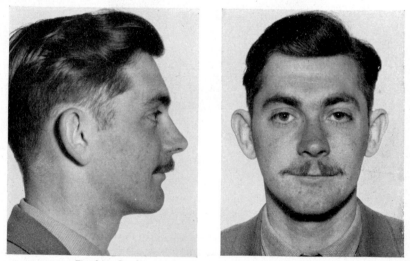

Fig. 34.—Profile and full face of patient shown in Fig. 32.

overcome in the Royal Berkshire Hospital halo (Mackenzie and Ray, 1970) which encircles three-quarters of the skull and leaves the occiput free. (*Fig.* 30.) However, it still interferes with the patient lying comfortably on his side and most patients find the plaster-of-Paris headcap more satisfactory when lying in bed.

The connexion between the upper jaw and the headcap is achieved by attaching a splint to the tooth-bearing portion of the upper and lower jaw and, after reducing the fracture, either the upper or the lower jaw is connected to the headcap by anterior connecting rods and possibly by transbuccal cheek wires.

If the patient has teeth, a silver/copper alloy cap splint is cemented over the upper and lower teeth, and if the patient is edentulous a Gunning type splint is wired to the jaws by peralveolar and circumferential wires.

To either the upper or lower splint, a projecting bar is attached in the incisor area.

Incorporated in the plaster-of-Paris headcap is a wire frame which projects anteriorly, and this is connected to the anterior projecting bar from the splints by an anterior connecting rod and universal joints. (*Fig.* 31.)

The upper splint has a hook on either side in the first molar region and when transbuccal cheek wires are used, they are fixed to these hooks and pass through the cheeks to be attached to the frame in the headcap. There is an attachment on the headcap frame which enables the transbuccal cheek wires to have their tension and direction of pull adjusted.

Immobilization achieved by connecting the upper jaw to the headcap is known as 'cranio-maxillary fixation'. This type of fixation enables the mandible to be freed so that the occlusion can be checked. (*Figs.* 32–34.)

When the lower jaw is immobilized to the headcap, it is referred to as 'cranio-mandibular fixation'. When this type of immobilization is used, the mandible cannot be released until treatment is completed, by which time it is impossible to alter the position of the upper jaw in order to adjust the occlusion.

Fractures in patients with a normal angle Class III occlusion require cranio-mandibular fixation, as it is difficult to fit an anterior connecting bar to the maxilla in such cases.

Cheek Wires: Transbuccal cheek wires are most helpful for elevating the tuberosity region of the tooth-bearing fragment during reduction, and, together with the anterior connecting rod, they provide a stable three-point fixation from the headcap. They are passed through the cheeks at a suitable point in line with the upper cap splint hooks and headcap attachments. Their passage through the tissues is effected by the use of a cannula such as a spinal needle or by using a long straight needle.

They are usually used in cranio-maxillary fixation, but they can be connected to circumferential wires in the mandible and this constitutes an efficient method of fixation of a middle-third fracture by sandwiching it between an intact mandible and a headcap.

Indications for the Use of Extra-oral Immobilization: Extra-oral immobilization by suspension from a plaster-of-Paris headcap is most commonly used in well-equipped maxillo-facial units where facilities for the construction of splints are available.

If splints cannot be provided, the fractured middle third of the facial skeleton may be sandwiched between the mandible and a headcap by attaching cheek wires from the headcap to circumferential wires in the lower canine region and mandibular-maxillary fixation is usually carried out by inter-dental eyelet wiring or with arch bars.

2. *Indirect Skeletal Fixation:*

a. Zygomatico-mandibular fixation is achieved by inserting one extra-oral pin into the mandible and zygomatic bone on each side and connecting them with rods and universal joints. This method can be used in Le Fort I and II type fractures.

The same effect can be achieved by transfixing the mandible and the zygomatic bones with Kirschner wires or Steinmann pins and connecting the upper and lower pins or wires with bars and universal joints.

b. Fronto-mandibular fixation is achieved by inserting pins into the mandible and connecting them by bars and universal joints to pins inserted in the frontal bone. This method is used in the treatment of Le Fort III fractures.

In both zygomatico-mandibular and fronto-mandibular fixation the fractured middle third is sandwiched between two stable parts of the facial skeleton, but this method can only be used when the molar teeth are intact.

Immobilization within the Tissues.—

These techniques require no special laboratory facilities for the construction of splints and, as none of the fixation is visible, the patients are not so conspicuous as with extra-oral immobilization, and may be discharged from hospital earlier. Fixation of the fractures from within the tissues is also an advantage when the patient is cerebrally irritated or mentally deranged and is therefore liable to tear off any extra-oral appliances.

1. *a. Direct fixation by transosseous wiring* at the zygomatico-maxillary and zygomatico-frontal fracture lines has been described in the section on zygomatic complex fractures, as has direct wiring of the comminuted zygomatic bone.

Midline splits of the palate may be immobilized by transosseous wiring.

b. Transfixation with Kirschner wires: Fixation of the middle-third fracture is achieved by inserting a Kirschner wire through the body of one zygomatic bone into the body of the zygomatic bone on the opposite side, so that the wire transfixes the maxillae and the nasal septum. A similar result can be produced by driving a Kirschner wire through each zygomatic bone and down into the nasal septum, the two wires transfixing the nasal septum from opposite sides.

These transfixation techniques produce a surprisingly rigid fixation and at the completion of treatment the wire can be removed under local analgesia. These wires pass through the maxillary sinuses and the nasal passages and, as infection may occur, antibiotic cover is advisable. This method is technically difficult, especially if one or more zygomatic bones are unstable, and great care is necessary to avoid damage to the eyes.

2. *Suspension by Wires from some Stable Portion of the Facial Skeleton above the Line of Fracture:* The suspension wires are connected to circumferential wires in the lower canine region, and the fractured middle third

is sandwiched between the mandible and the base of the skull. The wires are passed through the tissues with the aid of long curved needles, awls, or cannulas. The suspension may be:—

a. Circumzygomatic, when the wires pass over the zygomatic arch (*Fig.* 35).

b. Zygomatico-mandibular: The wire is passed through a small hole drilled in the body of the zygomatic bone, access being obtained through a small incision beneath the bone.

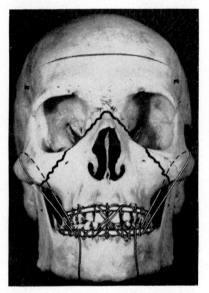

Fig. 35.—Diagram of circumzygomatic wiring. A wire is passed over the zygomatic arch and secured to an arch bar attached to the mandibular teeth. The fractured portion of the upper jaw is sandwiched between the mandible and the intact portion of the middle third of the facial skeleton.

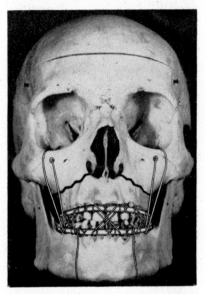

Fig. 36.—Diagram of a Le Fort I fracture immobilized by sandwiching the fractured area between the mandible and an intact portion of the middle third of the facial skeleton above the line of fracture. A small hole has been drilled through the inferior orbital rim, and a wire through this hole has been passed round an arch bar attached to the mandibular teeth.

c. Inferior orbital border-mandibular wiring is carried out by drilling a small hole through the lower border of the orbit, access being obtained through a 1-in. or 2·5 cm. semilunar incision beneath the orbit (*Fig.* 36).

d. Fronto-mandibular, by passing the wires through a hole in the *zygomatic process of the frontal bone,* the surgical approach being made through one of the wrinkles at the outer aspect of the orbit (*Figs.* 37, 39).

e. Pyriform fossa-mandibular wiring is only of value in treating Le Fort I type fractures. The pyriform fossa is approached by an incision in the buccal sulcus. A muco-periosteal flap is raised to expose the lateral bony wall of the nasal cavity in which a hole is drilled (*Fig.* 38).

f. Nasal septum-mandibular: A similar proceeding may be carried out using the nasal septum, but this fixation is not so stable as some of the other forms of suspension.

None of these suspension techniques produces an absolutely rigid fixation and some anteroposterior movements of the fragments are possible, but these are controlled by combining the suspension with mandibular-maxillary fixation by eyelet wiring or arch bars.

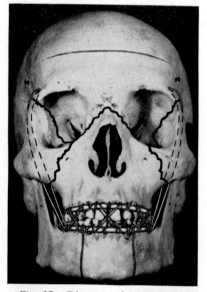

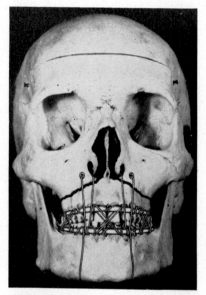

Fig. 37.—Diagram of a Le Fort III fracture immobilized by sandwiching the fractured area between the mandible and the base of the skull. A wire passing through a hole drilled in the zygomatic process of the frontal bone above the fracture line is attached to an arch bar on the mandibular teeth.

Fig. 38.—Diagram of a Le Fort type I fracture immobilized by sandwiching the fractured area between the mandible and the intact portion of the middle third of the facial skeleton above the fracture line. A wire through a hole drilled in the pyriform fossa area is connected to circumferential wires.

To facilitate removal of the wires when treatment is completed, the wires are passed through the holes and back into the mouth. Traction on the cut end of the wire in the mouth enables them to be pulled through.

In the more extensive type of fracture it may sometimes be necessary to carry out transosseous wiring at the zygomatico-frontal and zygomatico-maxillary fracture lines before a relatively fixed portion of the facial skeleton is available for immobilization by suspension.

The development of treatment by immobilization within the tissues by the use of wires and pins has been made possible by the use of antibiotics without which many of these wires, passing as they do through infected cavities such as the nares, mouth, and maxillary sinuses, would become infected.

3. *Support:*

a. Antral packs: The question of packs in the maxillary sinus to support a mobile zygomatic bone has been discussed in the section on zygomatic complex fractures.

b. Antral balloons: The use of antral balloons to support the zygomatic bone has been advocated (Jackson, Abbey, and Clauz, 1956). The balloon is inserted through an intranasal antrostomy and removed from the nose at the conclusion of treatment. The balloon has a stem which emerges from the nostril, and the balloon is inflated with a Luer-Lok syringe, after which the tube is plugged with a spigot.

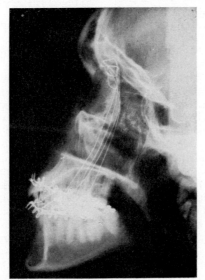

Fig. 39.—A lateral radiograph which depicts the suspension wires passing behind the zygomatic buttresses, and shows the circumferential wires below which secure the lower arch bar.

The use of the Foley catheter for the same purpose has been suggested by Walden and Bromberg (1957), who suggest filling the catheter with lipidol, and by Jarabak (1959).

CHOICE OF METHOD OF TREATMENT.—The type of fixation used in any particular middle-third injury must depend upon the nature of the fracture and the facilities available.

As a very general rule, extra-oral immobilization is used when the operator has at his disposal a well-equipped maxillo-facial laboratory, while immobilization within the tissues is favoured by surgeons working without these facilities. Extra-oral fixation produces a more rigid immobilization of the facial fractures.

Immobilization within the tissues holds the fragments upwards very effectively but there is a greater tendency for the bones of the middle of the face to be displaced backwards. In fact, the fronto-mandibular wires tend to pull the fractured portion of the facial bones distally.

Excellent results can be achieved with any of the methods of fixation already discussed, and the most important factor in the treating of these fractures is the careful reduction of the main fragments. It is not difficult to reposition the main tooth-bearing fragment in order to restore the occlusion, but the final result of the treatment depends to a considerable extent on the careful reduction of the zygomatic and nasal complexes to avoid an ugly residual flattening of the face.

OUTLINE OF DEFINITIVE PROCEDURES IN FACIAL FRACTURES WHERE TREATMENT HAS BEEN DELAYED

1. DENTO-ALVEOLAR FRACTURES.—Teeth which have been subjected to trauma frequently develop apical infection, and if they are seen on the first occasion a considerable time after injury they usually require extraction.

Alveolar fractures either unite in an incorrect position or give rise to infection and the fragments sequestrate.

Tooth or bone fragments in the lip either become infected or remain as hard lumps in the lip, which cause the patient considerable irritation. They can easily be removed from an intra-oral approach.

2. ZYGOMATIC COMPLEX FRACTURES.—If some two weeks are allowed to elapse before reducing a fractured zygomatic bone, the fracture will probably be unstable because the fractured ends will no longer interdigitate efficiently. This is due to osteoclastic activity rounding off the bony spicules and transosseous wiring or pinning will therefore be required. After about a month, it will be found almost impossible to elevate a fractured zygomatic bone in the conventional manner. If such a depressed zygomatic bone is causing diplopia or limitation of mandibular movements, re-fracture will be necessary. If the depression is merely causing a cosmetic deformity, an onlay graft of bone or cartilage will suffice. If interference with mandibular movement is the main symptom, a coronoidectomy on the affected side may be preferable to the more extensive surgery required to re-fracture and re-position the zygomatic bone.

Diplopia caused by enophthalmos due to orbital-floor fracture, as in the 'blow-out' syndrome, is difficult to treat. Bone-grafts or Teflon grafts beneath the globe of the eye combined with strabismus type operations may be necessary to correct the defect.

3. NASAL COMPLEX FRACTURES.—To obtain a satisfactory functional and aesthetically pleasing result it is essential that nasal fractures are treated soon after the injury. Neglected cases require nasal re-fracture and possibly a submucous resection of the septum. More severe cases require a bone-graft to the bridge and, if the entire naso-ethmoidal area is flattened, as in the 'dish-face' deformity, a post-nasal inlay may be required.

4. LE FORT I, II, AND III TYPE FRACTURES.—When treatment has not been unduly delayed, it may be possible to re-position the tooth-bearing portion of the upper jaw by fitting a splint to the teeth in the upper jaw and then pulling it upwards and forwards by attaching it to a 4-lb. weight via a cord over a pulley on a Balkan beam. This method is often effective if the fracture is not actually united. It will reduce the tooth-bearing portion of the fracture but do nothing to correct zygomatic and naso-ethmoidal complex fractures.

If union of the fragments has occurred, the fracture line can be exposed and re-fractured through an incision in the buccal sulcus, and the tooth-bearing portion can then be re-positioned.

In cases where lack of treatment has resulted in gagging of the bite in the molar area, grinding of the teeth or selective extraction and alveolec-tomy may enable an acceptable occlusion to be restored.

Treatment of the zygomatic complex and nasal complex areas will also be required.

The treatment of severe facial fractures which have been allowed to unite in malposition presents a very difficult problem in reconstructive surgery, and every effort should be made to effect reduction of such fractures before bony union occurs.

Post-operative Management of Fractures of the Middle Third of the Facial Skeleton

Immediate Post-operative Care.—At the conclusion of operation, a nasopharyngeal airway is inserted and it is kept patent by occasional aspiration with a length of $\frac{1}{8}$-in. or 3-mm. bore polythene tubing attached to a sucker nozzle.

If cranio-maxillary fixation has been employed, it is possible to defer maxillary-mandibular fixation until the patient has fully recovered consciousness to enable him to breathe through the mouth.

If the jaws are fixed together, a suture can be passed through the dorsum of the tongue and brought out of the mouth through the fixation to enable the tongue to be controlled while the patient is unconscious.

The patient should be nursed on the side to allow blood and saliva to dribble out of the mouth.

If extra-oral fixation has been employed, care should be taken to prevent the patient damaging the appliances during recovery from the anaesthetic. A suction apparatus, oxygen, tracheostomy set, wire cutters, and screw-drivers should be available at the patient's bedside in case an emergency should occur which necessitates the removal of the appliances.

The nasopharyngeal airways should be left in position until the patient is fully conscious and has an adequate airway.

No analgesics or hypnotics are given in the immediate post-operative phase, and morphine is especially contra-indicated as it depresses the cough reflex. If the patient is cerebrally irritated or restless, 3–8 ml. of paraldehyde are given intramuscularly.

An experienced nurse should be at the bedside until the patient has recovered consciousness.

Management after the Patient has recovered Consciousness.— The patient should be nursed in the sitting position to facilitate respiration, provided there is no contra-indication such as a fracture of the vertebrae.

Following the removal of the nasopharyngeal airway, respiration may be helped by occasional suction around the buccal sulcus. Clearing of blood and mucus from the teeth and coating the lips with petroleum jelly enables the patient to breathe comfortably through the mouth.

A 5-day course of intramuscular penicillin, 500,000 units b.d., should be given and if there is a cerebrospinal fluid leak, 1·0 g. of sulphatriad is given 6-hourly. If the patient cannot take sulphonamides by mouth, sulphadiazine should be given intramuscularly.

Adequate fluids by mouth are required and a fluid balance sheet is kept.

No analgesics or hypnotics are desirable or necessary, for if the fracture is adequately immobilized there is no pain.

An hourly pulse chart is kept until the clinician considers that it may be discontinued.

Rise in body temperature may be indicative of local infection in the fracture site or associated injury, or herald the onset of respiratory complications.

The patient should be visited by the clinician twice a day, and a careful watch is kept on the general condition.

Alterations in the patient's manner such as increased irritability should be noted as they may indicate the onset of some complication such as meningitis, intracranial haemorrhage or formation of an aerocoele.

Regular examinations of the chest are carried out, and the patient's legs should be examined for early signs of thrombophlebitis.

FEEDING.—Either a fluid or a semi-solid diet will be necessary, depending on the type of fixation employed, and patients have no difficulty in sucking the food through their oral fixation.

The semi-solid diet is produced by mincing the normal diet and passing it through a wire sieve of 16 meshes to the inch (2·5 cm.), after which it is mixed with soup. An electric food mixer with a liquidizer attachment is invaluable for this purpose. A feeding cup with a spout to which an 8-in. (or 20-cm.) length of rubber tubing is attached enables patients to feed themselves by passing the end of the rubber tubing through a gap in the fixation or round the back of the lower teeth in the retromolar fossa region. Flexible drinking straws such as Flex-Straw (manufactured by Sweetheart Bristol Ltd.) are also very helpful to enable a bed patient to drink from a vessel. The diet should be supplemented with vitamins.

Small quantities of fluid and semi-solid diets are very filling, and to give an adequate calorific intake the patient should be fed every 6 hours. Vary the menu as much as possible: Complan makes a valuable addition to the diet. A feeding cup with a length of rubber tube attached to the spout enables the patient to feed himself.

ORAL HYGIENE.—In the early stages irrigation of the mouth should be carried out after every meal, using a Higginson's syringe and warm 2 per cent sodium bicarbonate solution. Later the patient can clean the mouth and splints with a soft toothbrush.

LATE POST-OPERATIVE PHASE.—Early ambulation is desirable, and until this is possible the patient should have regular breathing and foot exercises.

Fractures are united in four to five weeks and fixation can be removed at this time. Patients should not be discharged from hospital with extra-oral fixation appliances in position, but can return home while their fractures are immobilized with fixation within the tissues, provided their general medical condition is satisfactory.

LATE COMPLICATIONS OF FRACTURES OF THE MIDDLE THIRD OF THE FACIAL SKELETON

If the patient has been adequately treated, there are surprisingly few late complications of the fracture, but often the patient has symptoms arising from the associated head injury.

COMPLICATIONS FROM THE HEAD INJURIES.—Most cases suffer to a greater or lesser extent from the post-concussional syndrome which consists of headache, dizziness, insomnia, diplopia, intolerance to noise, changes in disposition, intellectual impairment, and intolerance to alcohol. Usually these distressing symptoms eventually resolve, but may become aggravated and protracted if litigation for compensation is impending.

An aerocoele or a cerebral abscess may develop within a few weeks of the accident. Meningitis may occur as an early or a very late complication, and occasionally epilepsy develops.

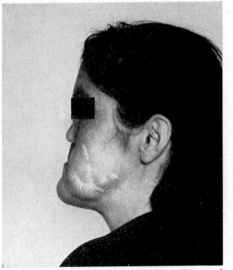

Fig. 40.—'Dish-face' deformity following a Le Fort III type fracture.

COMPLICATIONS ARISING FROM THE FRACTURE.—

1. If the fracture is inadequately reduced, there may be bony deformity of the face which consists of flattening of one or both zygomatic regions, flattening or deviation of the nose, or, in the untreated case, flattening of the entire face, producing the so-called 'dish-face' deformity (*Fig.* 40). Inadequately reduced fractures of Le Fort I, II, and III type show excessive lengthening of the face. There is gagging of the molar teeth with an anterior open bite, and, as the mandible is already pushed open by the upper jaw being too far down, the patient complains of being 'unable to open the mouth'.

2. There may be diplopia, enophthalmos, strabismus, alteration of the pupillary level, and, in exceptional cases, blindness.

3. Blockage of the nares by a deviated septum may prevent the patient from breathing through the nose.

4. Damage to the nasolacrimal duct may cause epiphora.

5. There may be anaesthesia in the distribution of one or both infra-orbital nerves.

6. There may be anaesthesia in the distribution of the fifth cranial nerve—usually involving the anterior, middle, and posterior superior dental nerves.

7. There may be anosmia due to damage to the olfactory nerve when the cribriform plate of the ethmoid is comminuted as in Le Fort II and III type and severe nasal complex fractures. This is a permanent disability.

8. There may be limitation of mandibular excursion due to the coronoid process impinging on a depressed zygomatic bone.

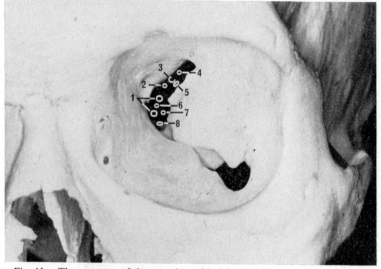

Fig. 41.—The contents of the superior orbital fissure.
1, The oculomotor nerve. 2, The trochlear nerve. 3, The frontal nerve. 4, The lacrimal nerve.   5, The superior ophthalmic vein.   6, The naso-ciliary nerve. 7, The abducent nerve. 8, The inferior ophthalmic vein.
In order to demonstrate the full extent of the superior orbital fissure, the photograph is angled so that the optic foramen is not shown.

9. Bony union occurs comparatively rapidly and non-union of fractures of the middle third of the facial skeleton is unknown, though occasionally there may be some slight spring in the upper jaw which may persist for some weeks.

10. *The Superior Orbital Fissure Syndrome.*—Fractures of the facial bones, particularly the zygomatic complex, may very rarely be complicated by damage to the contents of the superior orbital fissure (*Fig.* 41). The trauma may cause disruption of the bony margins of the fissure, or haematoma or aneurysm formation within the fissure may involve the 3rd, 4th and 6th cranial nerves. This results in ophthalmoplegia, ptosis, proptosis, and a fixed dilated pupil. The dilatation of the pupil is probably due to a parasympathetic block and the proptosis to paralysis of the extra-ocular muscles which normally exert a retracting force on the globe. There is a sensory disturbance over the distribution of the ophthalmic division of the 5th cranial nerve. The prognosis is poor when nerves have been traumatized, but in most cases there is a slow complete or partial recovery of the motor and sensory nerves involved.

BIBLIOGRAPHY

ADAMS, W. M. (1942), 'Internal Wiring Fixation of Facial Fractures', *Surgery*, **12**, 523.
— — and ADAMS, L. H. (1956), 'Internal Wire Fixation of Facial Fractures: A Fifteen-year Follow-up Report', *Amer. J. Surg.*, **92**, 12.
AKAMINE, R. N. (1955), 'Diagnosis of Traumatic Injuries of the Face and Jaws', *Oral Surg.*, **8**, 349.
ALBRIGHT, C. R. (1972), 'Management of Mid-facial Fractures', *Ibid.*, **34**, 858.
ALEXANDER, E., HARRILL, J. A., and SATTERWHITE, W. M. (1964), 'Skeletal Traction for Facial Fractures', *Surg. Gynec. Obstet.*, **119**, 1326.
ALLEN, N. E. (1957), 'Horizontal Fractures of the Maxilla and Compound Fractures of the Mandible', *Ibid.*, **10**, 345.
ALLING, C. C. (1959), 'Trends in Maxillofacial Surgery in Acute Trauma', *Ibid.*, **12**, 1387.
— — (1960), 'Early Management of Maxillofacial Mass Casualties', *J. oral Surg.*, **18**, 218.
ANDERSON, M. (1964), 'Blow-out Fractures', *Ibid.*, **22**, 405.
ARLOTTA, P., and PIZZONI, D. (1966), 'Fractures of the Zygomatic Complex', *Brit. J. oral Surg.*, **4**, 192.
ATIYEH, W. A., MAY, M., and GILDERSLEEVE, G. (1966), 'Acute True Blow-out Fracture of the Orbit', *Sth. med. J., Nashville*, **59**, 332.
BALASUBRAMANIAN, S. (1966), 'Intra-oral Approach for Reduction of Malar Fractures', *Brit. J. oral Surg.*, **4**, 189.
BANKS, P. (1967), 'Superior Orbital Fissure Syndrome', *Oral Surg.*, **24**, 455.
BARCLAY, T. L. (1960), 'Four Hundred Malar-zygomatic Fractures', *Trans. Int. Soc. plast. Surg.*, p. 259. Edinburgh: Livingstone.
BATTLE, R. J. V. (1953), 'War History of Plastic Surgery in the Army', *History of the Second World War (Surgery)*, p. 341. London: Her Majesty's Stationery Office.
BEYER, C. K. et al. (1971), 'Naso-orbital Fractures, Complications and Treatment', *Ophthalmologica*, **163**, 418.
BINGHAM, C. B. (1955), 'Fractured Malar', *Oral Surg.*, **8**, 13.
BLAIR, V. P., IVY, R. H., and BROWN, J. B. (1951), *Essentials of Oral Surgery*, 4th ed. London: Kimpton.
BONNETTE, G. H., and GARCIA-OLLER, J. L. (1957), 'Skull Tongs in Craniomaxillary Fixation: Report of a Case', *J. oral Surg.*, **15**, 156.
BOUDREAUX, R. E. (1957), 'Modified Metal Urethral Sound: A New Instrument in Reduction of Zygomatic Fractures', *Ibid.*, **15**, 31.
BRADLEY, J. L. (1956), 'Primary Treatment of Maxillofacial Injuries', *Oral Surg.*, **9**, 371.
— — and BONNETTE, G. H. (1955), 'Fractures of the Zygoma (Malar) Zygomatic Compound', *Ibid.*, **8**, 237.
BRITISH ASSOCIATION OF ORAL SURGEONS (1972), 'Symposium on Complications of Middle Third Fractures', *Brit. J. oral. Surg.*, **9**, 161.
BROWN, J. B., FRYER, M. P., and McDOWELL, F. (1949), 'Internal Wire Pin Immobilization of Jaw Fractures', *Plast. reconstr. Surg.*, **4**, 30.

BROWN, P. R. (1966), 'An Adjustable Method of Maxillary Traction for Fractures of the Central Middle Third of the Face', *Brit. J. oral Surg.*, **4,** 23.

BRYANT, F. L. (1960), 'Management of Maxillofacial Fractures', *Laryngoscope (St Louis)*, **70,** 647.

CAIRNS, H. (1937), 'Injuries of the Frontal and Ethmoidal Sinuses with Special Reference to Cerebrospinal Rhinorrhoea and Aeroceles', *J. Laryng.*, **52,** 589.

CALVERT, C. A. (1942), 'Discussion of Injuries of the Frontal and Ethmoidal Sinuses', *Proc. R. Soc. Med.*, **35,** 805.

CAPODANNO, J. (1967), 'Reconstruction of Acutely Traumatised Orbital Floor', *J. oral Surg.*, **25,** 510.

CARTER, W. S. (1970), 'Midfacial Trauma', *Nebraska Med. J.*, **55,** 220.

CHARLTON, H. (1967), 'An Occipital Air Support for Use with the Ellis "Halo" ', *Brit. J. oral Surg.*, **5,** 167.

CHRISTENSEN, E. W. (1962), 'Problems in the Management of Severe Maxillofacial Trauma', *J. Ky med. Ass.*, **60,** 155.

CLARKSON, P. W., WILSON, T. H. H., and LAWRIE, R. S. (1946), 'Treatment of 1,000 Jaw Fractures', *Brit. dent. J. (Services Suppl.)*, **77,** 229.

COHEN, B. M. (1958), 'Malar Fractures', *Oral Surg.*, **11,** 1081.

—— (1961), 'Multiple Facial Fractures', *Ibid.*, **14,** 129.

COHEN, L. (1960), 'Fractures of the Maxillary Tuberosity occurring during Tooth Extraction', *Ibid.*, **13,** 409.

CONVERSE, J. M. (1957), 'Enophthalmos and Diplopia in Fractures of the Orbital Floor', *Brit. J. plast. Surg.*, **41,** 265.

CONWAY, H. et al. (1970), 'Another Method of bringing the Midface Forward', *Plast. reconstr. Surg.*, **46,** 325.

CRAMER, L., TOOZE, F., and LERMAN, S. (1965), 'Blow-out Fractures of the Orbit', *Brit. J. plast. Surg.*, **18,** 171.

CRAWFORD, M. J. (1943), 'Appliances and Attachments for Treatment of Upper Jaw Fractures', *Nav. med. Bull.*, **41,** 1151.

CREWE, T. C. (1966), 'A Halo Frame for Facial Injuries', *Brit. J. oral Surg.*, **4,** 147.

CRIKELAIR, G. F. et al. (1972), 'A Critical Look at the "Blow-out", Fracture', *Plast. reconstr. Surg.*, **49,** 374.

CROWE, W. W. (1959), 'Treatment of Zygomatic Fractures-Dislocations" *J. oral Surg.*, **17,** 27.

CUTRIGHT, D. E. et al. (1972), 'The Repair of Fractures of the Orbital Floor using Biodegradable Polylactic Acid', *Oral Surg.*, **33,** 28.

DANDY, (1945), 'Diagnosis and Treatment of Strictures of Aquaduct of Sylvius', *Arch. Surg.*, **57,** 1.

DAVIES, A. S. (1972), 'Traumatic Defects of the Orbital Floor', *Brit. J. oral Surg.*, **10,** 133.

DAWSON, R. L. (1957), 'The Four Screw Maxillary Fixation', *Brit. J. plast. Surg.*, **9,** 311.

—— and FORDYCE, G. L. (1953), 'Complex Fractures of the Middle Third of the Face and their Early Treatment', *Brit. J. Surg.*, **41,** 255.

DINGMAN, R. O. and NATVIG, P. (1964), *Surgery of Facial Fractures.* London: Saunders.

DONALDSON, K. I. (1961), 'Fractures of the Facial Skeleton: A Survey of 335 Patients', *N.Z. dent. J.*, **57**, 55.

EDWARDS, J. (1964), 'A Modified Technique for the Placement of Circumzygomatic Wires', *Brit. J. oral Surg.*, **2**, 205.

ELLEGAST, H. H. et al. (1972), 'The Radiological Management of Blow-out Fractures', *Dentomaxillofac. Radiol.*, **1**, 45.

EMERY, J. M. et al. (1972), 'Management of Orbital Floor Fractures', *Amer. J. Ophthal.*, **74**, 299.

EVANS, J. N. G., and FENTON, P. J. (1971), 'Blow-out Fracture of the Orbit', *J. Laryngol. Otol.*, **85**, 1127.

FICKLING, B. W. (1946), 'Advances in Construction and Use of Splints in Treatment', *Brit. dent. J.*, **80**, 8.

FREEMAN, B. S. (1962), 'The Direct Approach to Acute Fractures of the Zygomatico-maxillary Complex and Immediate Prosthetic Replacement of the Orbital Floor', *Plast. reconstr. Surg.*, **29**, 587.

FRY, W. K., SHEPHERD, P. P., MCLEOD, A. C., and PARFITT, G. J. (1943), *The Dental Treatment of Maxillofacial Injuries.* Oxford: Blackwell.

FRYER, M. P., and BROWN, J. B. (1955), 'Multiple Internal Wire Fixation of Facial Fractures', *Amer. J. Surg.*, **89**, 814.

—— et al. (1972), 'Repair of Trauma about the Orbit', *J. Trauma*, **12**, 290.

FUNK, E. C. (1961), 'Emergency Treatment of Maxillofacial Injuries', *Int. dent. J.*, **10**, 476.

GEORGIADE, N. G. (1972), 'The Management of Acute Mid-facial Orbital Injuries', *Clin. Neurosurg.*, **19**, 301.

GILLIES, H. D., KILNER, T. P., and STONE, D. (1927), 'Fractures of the Malar Zygomatic Compound with a Description of a New X-ray Position', *Brit. J. Surg.*, **14**, 651.

GOLDBERG, M. G., and WILLIAMS A. C. (1969),' The Location and Occurrence of Mandibular Fractures. An Analysis of 202 Cases.' *Oral Surg.*, **28**, 336.

GOLDMAN, I. B. (1961), 'Middle Third Facial Fracture Complications', *Eye, Ear, Nose, Thr. Monthly*, **40**, 356.

GOLDMAN, R. J. et al. (1973), 'Appraisal of Surgical Correction in 130 Cases of Orbital Floor Fracture', *Amer. J. Ophthal.*, **76**, 152.

GORDON, S. (1957), 'Malar Fracture: Intra-orbital Haemorrhage during Open Reduction', *Plast. reconstr. Surg.*, **20**, 65.

GUTMAN, B. S., LAUFER, D., and NEDER, A. (1964), 'The Use of the Foley Catheter in the Treatment of Zygomatic Bone Fractures', *Brit. J. oral Surg.*, **2**, 153.

HARNISCH, H. (1960), 'Five-year Statistics of Jaw Fractures', *Zahnärztl. Prax.*, **10**, 126.

HARRIS, H. H. (1958), 'Fixation of Fractures in the Middle Third of the Face with Kirschner Wires', *Laryngoscope (St Louis)*, **68**, 95.

HAVERLING, M. (1972), 'Diagnosis of Blow-out Fractures of the Orbit by Tomography', *Acta Radiol.*, **12**, 347.

HAYTON-WILLIAMS, D. S. (1961), 'Skeletal Traction for Maxillary Fracture', *Oral Surg.*, **14**, 648.

HESLOP, I. (1964), 'Complicated Maxillofacial Injuries', *J. oral Surg.*, **22**, 151.

HIGHTOWER, D. R. et al. (1971), 'Current Concepts in the Treatment of Fractures of the Orbit', *Laryngoscope (St Louis)*, **81**, 725.

HOLLAND, N. W. A. (1945), 'The Use of Cheek Wires in the Treatment of Fractures of the Maxilla', *Brit. dent. J.*, **79**, 333.

HOTTE, H. (1970), *Orbital Fractures*. London: Heinemann Medical Books.

HUT, M. (1960), 'Methods and Appliances for the Reduction and Fixation of Fractures of the Facial Bones', *Int. dent. J.*, **10**, 468.

IVY, R. H., and CURTIS, L. (1931), 'Fractures of the Upper Jaw and Malar Bone', *Ann. Surg.*, **94**, 337.

JACKSON, V. R., ABBEY, J. A., and CLAUZ, S., (1956), 'Balloon Technique for Treatment of Fractures of the Zygomatic Bone', *J. oral Surg.*, **14**, 14.

JAMES, W. W., and FICKLING, B. W. (1940), *Injuries of Face and Jaws.* London: Bale & Staples.

JARABAK, J. P. (1959), 'Use of the Foley Catheter in Supporting Zygomatic Fractures', *J. oral Surg. Anesth.*, **17**, 39.

KAZANJIAN, V. H. (1927), 'Treatment of Injuries of the Upper Part of the Face', *J. Amer. dent. Ass.*, **14**, 1607.

— — (1958), 'Observations in the Treatment of Deformities and Injuries of the Facial Bones during the Last 50 Years', *Mass. dent. Soc. J.*, **7**, 9.

— — and CONVERSE, J. M. (1949), *The Surgical Treatment of Facial Fractures*. Baltimore: Williams & Wilkins.

KELLY, D. E., and HARRIGAN, W. F. (1975), 'A Survey of Facial Fractures: Bellevue Hospital, 1948–1974'. *J. oral Surg.*, **33**, 146–149.

KING, E. F., and SAMUEL, E. (1944), 'Fractures of Orbit', *Trans. Ophthal. Soc. U.K.*, **64**, 134.

KNIGHT, J. S., and NORTH, J. F. (1961), 'The Classification of Malar Fractures: An Analysis of Displacement as a Guide to Treatment', *Brit. J. plast. Surg.*, **13**, 325.

KREIRLER, J. F., and KOCH, H. (1975), 'Endoscopic Findings of the Maxillary Sinus after Middle Face Fractures'. *J. Maxillo-facial Surgery*, **3**, 10–14.

KULOWSKI, J. (1956), 'Facial Injuries: A Common Denominator of Automobile Casualties', *J. Amer. dent. Ass.*, **53**, 32.

LE FORT, R. (1901), 'Etude Expérimentale sur les Fractures de la Machôire Supérieure', *Revue Chir.*, **23**, 208.

LEONE, C. R. (1972), 'Orbital Fractures', *Amer. Fam. Physician*, **5**, 102.

— — et al. (1972), 'Bilateral Blow-out Fractures', *Ann. Ophthal.*, **4**, 495.

LESNEY, T. A. (1956), 'Considerations in Diagnosis of Maxillary Fractures', *J. oral Surg.*, **14**, 137.

LEVIN, I. S. (1959), 'Surgical Treatment of Multiple Facial Fractures: Report of Three Cases', *Oral Surg.*, **12**, 657.

— — and BAADE, E. A. (1958), 'Surgical Treatment of Extensive Maxillo-facial Fractures: Report of a Case', *Ibid.*, **11**, 235.

LEWIN, W., and CAIRNS, H. (1951), 'Fractures of the Sphenoidal Sinus with Cerebrospinal Fluid Rhinorrhoea', *Brit. med. J.*, **1**, 1.

LEWIS, G. K. (1957), 'Fractures of the Upper and Lower Jaws', *J. int. Coll. Surg.*, **27**, 305.

LINDSTROM, D. (1960), 'Comparative Survey of Jaw Fractures during the Years 1948–1958', *Dent. Abstr., Chicago*, **5**, 596.

LIPMAN, J. S., et al. (1967), 'Traumatic Emphysema of Face and Neck associated with Mid-facial Fracture', *Oral Surg.*, **23**, 717.

LUNDQVIST, C. (1960), 'Emergency Treatment of Maxillofacial Injuries', *Int. dent. J.*, **10**, 476.

McCOY, F. J., CHANDLER, R. A., MAGNAN, C. G., MOORE, J. R., and SIEMSEN, G. (1962), 'An Analysis of Facial Fractures and their Complications', *Plast. reconstr. Surg.*, **29**, 381.

McINDOE, A. H. (1941), 'Surgical and Dental Treatment of Fractures of the Upper and Lower Jaw in Wartime', *Proc. R. Soc. Med.*, **34**, 267.

— — (1941), 'Diagnosis and Treatment of Injuries of the Middle Third of the Face', *Brit. dent. J.*, **71**, 235.

MACKENZIE, D. L., and RAY, K. R. (1970), 'The Royal Berkshire Hospital "Halo" ', *Brit. J. oral Surg.*, **8**, 27.

MAGNUS, W. W. (1971), 'A Conjunctival Approach to Repair of Fracture of Medial Wall of Orbit: Report of Case', *J. Oral Surg.*, **29**, 664.

MALLETT, S. P. (1950), 'Fractures of the Jaw: A Survey of 2124 Cases', *J. Amer. dent. Ass. dent. Cosmos*, **41**, 657.

MANSFIELD, O. T. (1948), 'Fractures of the Malazygomatic Compound', *Brit. J. plast. Surg.*, **1**, 123.

MARK, H. I. (1961), 'Reduction of a Zygomaticomaxillary Complex Fracture by the Antral Balloon Technique', *Oral Surg.*, **14**, 753.

MARONNEAUD, P. L. et al. (1959), 'Traumatic Lesions of the Upper Face in connection with Traffic Accidents. Statistical Study of 367 Cases of Fractures', *Toulouse Méd.*, **61**, 189.

MARTIN, B. C., TRABUE, J. C., and LEECH, T. R. (1956), 'An Analysis of the Etiology, Treatment and Complications of Fractures of the Malar Compound and Zygomatic Arch,' *Amer. J. Surg.*, **92**, 920.

MEREDITH, J. M. (1951), 'Surgical Aspects of Acute Head Injuries', *Surg. Gynec. Obstet.*, **93**, 3.

MILAUSKAS, A. T. (1969), *Blow-out Fractures of the Orbit*. Springfield, Ill.: Thomas.

— — and FUEGER, G. F. (1966), 'Serious Ocular Complications associated with Blow-out Fractures of the Orbit', *Amer. J. Ophthal.*, **62**, 670.

MILLER, S. H. et al. (1972), 'Current Concepts in the Diagnosis and Management of Fractures in the Orbital Floor', *Amer. J. Surg.*, **123**, 560.

MOHNAC, A. (1967), 'Maxillary Osteotomy for the Correction of Malpositioned Fractures', *J. oral Surg.*, **25**, 460.

MONTGOMERY, W. W. (1972), 'Facial Fractures related to the Orbit', *Laryngoscope (St Louis)*, **82**, 1897.

MORGAN, B. D. et al. (1972), 'Fractures of the Middle Third of the Face: A Review of 300 Cases', *Brit. J. plast. Surg.*, **25**, 147.

MUELLER, C. F. (1971), 'Blow-out Fracture of the Orbit', *Med. Trial. Tech. Quart.*, 388.

NEGUS, V. E. (1942), 'Discussion on Injuries of the Nose and Throat', *Proc. R. Soc. Med.*, **35**, 513.

NYSINGH, J. G. (1960), 'Zygomaticomaxillary Fractures with a Report of 200 Cases', *Arch. Chir. Neérl.*, **12**, 157.

OLDFIELD, M. C., and ROBERTS, W. R. (1947), 'Splints for Fractured Noses', *Brit. med. J.*, **1**, 886.

PANAGOPOULOS, A. P. (1959), 'Circumferential Wiring as an Aid to the Management of Maxillofacial Injuries', *J. int. Coll. Surg.*, **32**, 405.

PANUSKA, H. J., and DEDOLPH, T. H. (1965), 'Extra-oral Traction with Halo Head Frame for Complex Fractures ', *J. oral Surg.*, **23**, 212.

PELZER, R. H., and GARVIN, W. J. (1958), 'Controlled Correction of Diplopia and Eye Muscle Imbalance in Orbital and Zygomatic Fractures', *Amer. J. Surg.*, **96**, 735.

PERCY, E. C. (1971), 'Orbital Facial Fracture', *Can. med. Ass. J.*, **105**, 971.

PERRY, J. P., and NICKEL, V. L. (1959), 'Total Cervical Spine Fusion for Neck Paralysis', *J. Bone Jt Surg.*, **41-A**, 37.

PFEIFFER, R. (1943), 'Traumatic Enophthalmos'. *Arch. Ophth.*, **30**, 718.

PICKARD, B. H. et al. (1971), 'Fractures of the Ethmoid involving the Orbit', *Trans. ophthal. Soc. U.K.*, **91**, 515.

PIGGOT, T. A., and IRVING, M. (1966), ' Ophthalmoplegia in Fractures of the Malar Complex', *Brit. J. plast. Surg.*, **19**, 264.

PYBUS, P. K. (1971), 'A New Method for the Le Fort Type III Fractures of the Maxilla', *S. Afr. med. J.*, **45**, 991.

QUINN, J. (1968), ' Open Reduction and Internal Fixation of Vertical Maxillary Fractures ', *J. oral Surg.*, **26**, 167.

RABUZZI, D. D. (1971), 'Mid-facial Fractures', *N.Y. St. J. Med.*, **71**, 2412.

RASMUSSEN, K., and SCHLEGEL, C. (1958), 'Primary Operation in Zygomaticomaxillary Fractures with Diplopia', *Acta ophthal. (Kbh.)*, **36**, 468.

RICKER, O. L. (1962), 'Techniques of Internal Suspension of Maxillary Fractures', *J. oral Surg.*, **20**, 108.

ROBERTSON, D. C. (1956), 'The Treatment of Multiple Facial Fractures and Craniofacial Separation in the Patient with Concomitant Injuries', *Plast. reconstr. Surg.*, **18**, 367.

ROGERS, R. et al. (1972), 'Carotid Cavernous Sinus Fistula accompanying Mid-facial Fractures: Report of a Case', *J. oral Surg.*, **30**, 429.

ROWBOTHAM, G. F. (1949), *Acute Injuries of the Head*, 3rd ed. Edinburgh: Livingstone.

ROWE, N. L. (1964), ' First Aid Treatment, Diagnosis and Roentgenography of Maxillo-facial Injuries ', *J. oral Surg.*, **22**, 202.

— — (1973), 'Fractures of the Orbital Floor'. *Oral Surgery: Transactions of the 4th International Conference on Oral Surgery, Amsterdam, 1971*, p. 302. Copenhagen: Munksgaard.

— — and KILLEY, H. C. (1952), 'Fractures of the Facial Skeleton', *Dent. Practit.*, **3**, 34, 66.

— — — — (1968), *Fractures of the Facial Skeleton*, 2nd ed. Edinburgh: Livingstone.

RUMELT, M. B. et al. (1972), 'Isolated Blow-out Fracture of the Medial Orbital Wall with Medial Rectus Muscle Entrapment', *Amer. J. Ophthal.*, **73**, 451.

SABISTON, D. W. (1971), 'Management of Fractures of the Orbit', *Trans. Aust. Coll. Ophthal.*, **3**, 147.

SCHUCHARDT, K., SCHWENZER, N., ROTTKE, B., and LENTRODT, J. (1966), 'Ursachen Häufigkeit und Lokalisation der Frakturen des Gesichtes-schädels', *Fortschr. Kiefer. -u. Gesicht-Chir.*, **11**, 1.

SCHURTER, M., and LETTERMAN, G. S. (1956), 'Fractures of the Nose', *Post Grad. med. J.*, **19**, 354.

SHANDS, R. E. (1956), 'The Use of Transmaxillary Bar in Fractures of the Maxilla', *Amer. J. Surg.*, **91**, 106.

SHEPHERD, N. J. et al. (1971), 'Radiographic Evaluation of Lateral Orbital Rim', *Oral Surg.*, **32**, 494.

SHERMAN, M. J. (1955), 'Intra-oral Reduction of Maxillary Fractures by Malar Suspension', *J. oral Surg.*, **13**, 321.

SINGER, J. A. et al. (1970), 'Blow-out Fractures of the Orbit', *Nebraska med. J.*, **55**, 352.

SMALL, I. A., SIMMONS, D. R., and GASS, H. H. (1957), 'Fracture of the External Angular Process of the Frontal Bone: Its Relation to Maxillo-facial Fractures', *Ibid.*, **15**, 271.

SMILER, D. G. et al. (1971), 'Signs and Symptoms of Zygomatico-maxillary Fractures involving the Orbit', *J. oral Surg.*, **29**, 103.

SMITH, B. and REGAN, W. F. (1957), 'Blow-out Fracture of the Orbit', *Amer. J. Ophthal.*, **44**, 733.

— — et al. (1973), 'Differential Diagnosis in Orbital Injury: Internal Carotid-cavernous Sinus Fistula, Orbital Haematoma, Blow-out Fracture', *Archs Ophthal., Chicago*, **89**, 484.

SMITH, H. W. (1973), 'Pitfalls in the Treatment of Mid-facial Trauma', (Symposium on Maxillo-facial Trauma, IV), *Laryngoscope, St Louis*, **83**, 547.

— — and YANAGISAWA, E. (1961), 'Fracture Dislocations of Zygoma and Zygomatic Arch. Historical Development of Surgical Treatment', *Arch. Otolaryng.*, **73**, 172.

SNOW, J. B. (1972), 'The Management of Orbital Wall Fractures', *Trans. Amer. Acad. Ophthal. Otolaryngol.*, **74**, 1045.

STOCKDALE, C. R. (1958), 'Surgical Emphysema of the Face following a Middle Third Fracture', *Oral Surg.*, **11**, 135.

— — (1959), *Brit. J. plast. Surg.*, **12**, 78.

STOKES, R. F. (1956), 'Complication of Facial Bone Fractures', *Plast. reconstr. Surg.*, **17**, 73.

STUTEVILLE, O. H. (1956), 'The Surgical Treatment of Acute Injuries to the Soft Tissues and Bony Structures of the Face', *Amer. J. Surg.*, **92**, 864.

SVEINSSON, E. (1973), 'Pure Blow-out Fractures of the Orbital Floor', *J. Lar. Otol.*, **87**, 465.

TEBO, H. G. (1958), 'Personality Characteristics of Patients Treated in a Veterans Administration Hospital for Fracture of the Maxilla and Mandible', *Oral Surg.*, **11**, 681.

TEMPEST, M. (1960), 'The Surgical Management of Displaced Fractures of the Malar Bone', *Trans. Int. Soc. plast. Surg.*, p. 251. Edinburgh: Livingstone.

TESSIER, P. (1971), 'Total Osteotomy of the Middle Third of the Face for Faciostenosis or for Sequelae of Le Fort III Fractures', *Plastic reconstr. Surg.*, **48**, 533.

THOMA, K. H. (1942), *Traumatic Surgery of the Jaws*. St. Louis: Mosby.

THOMPSON, H. (1962), ' The "Halo" Traction Apparatus: A Method of External Splinting of the Cervical Spine after Injury', *J. Bone Jt Surg.*, **44-B**, 655.

TRAIGER, J. (1961), 'Fractures of the Maxillary Tuberosity occurring during Tooth Extraction involving the Maxillary Antrum', *Oral Surg.*, **14**, 246.

VAN HERK, W., and HOVINGA, J. (1973), 'Choice of Treatment of Orbital Floor Fractures as Part of Facial Fractures', *J. oral Surg.*, **31**, 600.

VIGARIO, G. D. (1967), 'A Radiological Analysis of 35 Cases of Blow-out Fractures of the Orbit', *Milit. Med.*, **132**, 545.

VOREAUX, M. P., and KNEIP, M. L. (1962), 'Treatment of Fractures of the Middle Third of the Face', *Dent. Abstr.*, **7**, 165.

WALDEN, R. H., and BROMBERG, B. E. (1957), 'Recent Advances in Therapy in Maxillofacial Bony Injuries in over 1000 Cases', *Amer. J. Surg.*, **93**, 508.

— — WOHLGEMUTH, P. R., and FITZ-GIBBON, J. H. (1956), 'Fractures of the Facial Bones', *Ibid.*, **92**, 915.

WALKER, G., HARRIGAN, W., ROWE, N. L., and WALKER, R. (1969), 'Clinical Pathological Conference on Facial Trauma', *J. oral Surg.*, **27**, 575.

WALTER, W. L. (1972), 'Early Surgical Repair of Blow-out Fracture of the Orbital Floor using the Transantral Approach', *Sth. med. J., Nashville*, **65**, 1229.

WARSON, R. W. (1971), 'Pseudo Ankylosis of the Mandible after a Fracture of the Zygomatico Maxillary Complex: Report of a Case', *J. oral Surg.*, **29**, 223.

WIESENBAUGH, J. (1970), 'Diagnostic Evaluation of Zygomatic Complex Fractures', *Ibid.*, **28**, 204.

YANAGISAW, E. (1973), 'Pitfalls in the Management of Zygomatic Fractures', (Symposium on Maxillo-facial Trauma, III), *Laryngoscope (St Louis)*, **83**, 527.

INDEX

Abscess, cerebral, as late complication in middle-third fractures, 75
Aerocoele, as late complication in middle-third fractures, 74, 75
Airway(s), ensuring patency of, 14, (*Figs*. 8, 9) 20–22
— nasal, involvement in maxillo-facial injuries, 9
— nasopharyngeal, use of, (*Fig*. 9) 21–22
Alveolar fractures (*see also* Dento-alveolar), definitive treatment, (*Fig*. 20) 52–53
Amnesia, 25
Analgesics, contra-indications for, 23–24, 73, 74
Anosmia, 76

Blindness following middle-third fractures, 75
Blood transfusions, 22

Cerebral irritation in middle-third fractures, 23
Cerebrospinal fluid rhinorrhoea, 48–49
— — — arresting, 49
— — — chemotherapy for, 23, 49, 73–74
— — — incidence, onset and duration, 48
— — — in Le Fort II fractures, 14, 43
— — — — III fractures, 14, 44
— — — meningitis following, 23, 49, 74–75
— — — in nasal complex fractures, 38, 39
— — — recording, 25
— — — testing for, 48
Classification of middle-third fractures, (*Figs*. 5–7) 16–19
Concussion, effects in middle-third fractures, 75

Dento-alveolar fractures (*see also* Middle-third fractures *and individual headings*), defined, (*Fig*. 6) 18, 19
— — definitive treatment, 51–53
— — — — where treatment delayed, 72
— — signs and symptoms, (*Fig*. 10) 27–28
— — — — clinical examination, 28
Dentures, removal, in immediate treatment procedures, 22
Dilated pupil, fixed, in superior orbital fissure syndrome, 76
Diplopia, 14, 26, 75
— in Le Fort II fractures, 42
— — — III fractures, 44
— orbital floor fractures, 37, 57

Diplopia, in zygomatic complex fractures, 32, 53–54, 72
'Dish-face' deformity, 72, (*Fig*. 40) 75

Ecchymosis, 25
— in isolated orbital floor fractures, 37
— Le Fort II fractures, 41–42
— — — III fractures, 44
— nasal complex fractures, 39
— zygomatic complex fractures, 31–33
Enophthalmos, 14, 75
— in Le Fort II fractures, 42
— — — III fractures, 44
— orbital floor fractures, 37, 57
— zygomatic complex fractures, 32
Epilepsy as late complication in middle-third fractures, 75
Epiphora, 15, 75
Epistaxis in isolated orbital floor fractures, 37
— nasal complex fractures, 39
— zygomatic complex fractures, 32
Ethmoid bone, comminution in middle-third fractures, (*Fig*. 4) 14
Eyes, involvement in maxillo-facial injuries, 9, 14

Feeding in post-operative management of middle-third fractures, 74
'Floaters', 41

Guérin type fractures, *see* Le Fort I type

Haemorrhage, 22, 25
— intracranial, as complication in middle-third fractures, 74
— — in Le Fort II fractures, 42
High-level fractures, *see* Le Fort III type
Hypnotics, contra-indications for, 23–24, 73, 74

Infra-zygomatic fractures, *see* Le Fort II type
Isolated orbital floor fractures, *see* Orbital floor fractures

Le Fort I type fractures (*see also* Middle-third fractures), definitive treatment, immobilization, (*Figs*. 36, 38) 62–72
— — — — — — — reduction, 60–61
— — — — — — — where treatment delayed, 72

Le Fort I type fractures described, (*Figs.* 5, 6) 16, 18
— — — — ensuring patency of airway in, (*Fig.* 8) 20
— — — — signs and symptoms, 40–42
— — — — unilateral, 47
— — II type fractures (*see also* Middle-third fractures), comminution of bone in, (*Figs.* 2–4) 14
— — — — definitive treatment, immobilization, 62–72
— — — — — — reduction, (*Fig.* 26) 61
— — — — — where treatment delayed, 72
— — — — described, (*Figs.* 5, 6) 16, 18
— — — — ensuring patency of airway in, (*Fig.* 8) 20, 21
— — — — maxillary sinuses involved, 15
— — — — nasolacrimal duct involved, 15
— — — — signs and symptoms, 41–44
— — — — — summarized, 43–44
— — — — superficial similarities to Le Fort III type, (*Fig.* 17) 41, 44
— — — — unilateral, 47
— — III type fractures (*see also* Middle-third fractures) associated with zygomatic complex fractures, 30
— — — — coexistent Le Fort I and II fractures in, 45, 46
— — — — comminution of bone in, (*Figs.* 2–4), 9, 14
— — — — definitive treatment, immobilization, (*Figs.* 27–35, 37, 39) 62–72
— — — — — reduction, 61–62
— — — — — where treatment delayed, 72–73
— — — — described, (*Figs.* 5–6) 16, 19
— — — — ensuring patency of airway in, (*Figs.* 8, 9) 20, 21
— — — — maxillary sinuses involved, 15
— — — — nasolacrimal duct involved, 15
— — — — signs and symptoms, 44–47
— — — — — summarized, 46–47
— — — — superficial similarities to Le Fort II type, (*Fig.* 17) 41, 44
— — — — unilateral, 47
'Loose faces', 41
Low-level fractures, *see* Le Fort II type

Mandibular closure, prevention of, (*Figs.* 2, 3) 15
Maxillae, separation of, 15

Maxillo-facial injuries (*see also* Middle-third fractures *and individual headings*), 9
— — incidence, 9–10
— — tissues and neighbouring structures involved, 9
Meningitis as complication in middle-third fractures, 23, 49, 74, 75
Middle third of facial skeleton, defined, 11–12
— — — — surgical anatomy of, (*Figs.* 1–4) 11–15
Middle-third fractures (*see also* Maxillo-facial injuries *and individual headings*), aetiology, 10
— — amnesia in, 25
— — cerebral irritation in, 23
— — cerebrospinal fluid rhinorrhoea in, *see* Cerebrospinal fluid rhinorrhoea
— — classification, (*Figs.* 5–7) 16–19
— — clinical examination, local, 25–26
— — — findings in, (*Figs.* 10–19) 27–47
— — defined, 9
— — history and description of symptoms, 25
— — incidence, 9–10
— — involving teeth and alveolus, (*Figs.* 6–7) 18–19
— — late complications of, (*Fig.* 40) 74–76
— — management, analgesics, contra-indications for, 23–24
— — — general medical examination, 23
— — — immediate treatment, (*Figs.* 8, 9) 20–22
— — — morphine contra-indicated, 23
— — — penicillin in, 23, 24, 73–74
— — — post-operative, 73–74
— — — preliminary examination, 22–24
— — — sulphonamides in, 23, 49, 73–74
— — not involving teeth and alveolus, (*Fig.* 7) 16–17
— — pain in, 23, 25, 74
— — relative frequency of types, (*Table I*) 19
Morphine contra-indicated in middle-third fractures, 23

Nares, blockage of, 14, 15, 21, 38, 43, 44, 48, 75
Nasal complex fractures (*see also* Middle-third fractures), comminution of bone in, (*Fig.* 4) 14
— — — defined, (*Fig.* 7) 16, 19
— — — definitive treatment, reduction, (*Fig.* 23) 58–59
— — — — splint fixation in, (*Figs.* 24–25) 59–60
— — — — where treatment delayed, 72
— — — ensuring patency of airway in, 21

Nasal complex fractures, nasolacrimal duct involved, 15
— — — signs and symptoms, 39–40
— — — surgical anatomy of, (*Figs.* 15–16) 38–39
Nasolacrimal duct, middle-third fractures involving, 15
Nerve(s), cranial, in middle-third fractures, (*Fig.* 41) 76
— dental, in middle-third fractures, 14, 76
— — zygomatic complex fractures, 33
— infra-orbital, in Le Fort III fractures, 45
— — middle-third fractures, 14, 75
— — zygomatic complex fractures, 32
— optic, in Le Fort II fractures, 42
— — middle-third fractures, 15

Oedema, 25
— in isolated orbital floor fractures, 37
— Le Fort II fractures, (*Fig.* 17) 41, 43
— — — III fractures, (*Fig.* 17) 41, 44, 45
— zygomatic arch fractures, 35
— — complex fractures, 31
Ophthalmoplegia in superior orbital fissure syndrome, 76
Orbit, middle-third fractures involving, 14
Orbital 'blow-in' fractures, 36–37
— 'blow-out' fractures, 36–37
— floor, comminution, in zygomatic complex fractures, 30
— — fractures, isolated, 36–38
— — — — applied surgical anatomy of, 36–37
— — — — definitive treatment, 57–58
— — — — diagnosis from entrapment of inferior oblique muscle, 37–38
— — — — radiology, 38
— — — — signs and symptoms, 37–38

Pain in middle-third fractures, 23, 25, 74
Penicillin, 23, 24, 73–74
Post-operative management of middle-third fractures, 73–74
Proptosis in isolated orbital floor fractures, 37
— superior orbital fissure syndrome, 76
Ptosis in superior orbital fissure syndrome, 76
Pyramidal type fractures, *see* Le Fort II type

Radiographs in dento-alveolar fractures, 27, 28

Radiology for middle-third fractures, 50
Road traffic accidents, principal cause of middle-third fractures, 10

Shock in middle-third fractures, 22
Sinuses, maxillary, middle-third fractures involving, 15
— paranasal, involvement in maxillo-facial injuries, 9
Strabismus as late complication in middle-third fractures, 75
— in Le Fort III fractures, 44
Sub-zygomatic fractures, *see* Le Fort II type
Sulphonamides, 23–24, 49, 73–74
Superior orbital fissure syndrome, (*Fig.* 41) 76
Supra-zygomatic fractures, *see* Le Fort III type

Teeth, avulsed, fractured or subluxated, 22, 27–28
— — definitive treatment, 51–52
Tongue, involvement in maxillo-facial injuries, 9
Tracheostomy, indications for, 22
Trismus, (*Figs.* 2, 3) 13, 41

Zygomatic arch fractures (*see also* Zygomatic complex fractures), (*Figs.* 12–14) 34–36
— — — definitive treatment, 56
— complex fractures (*see also* Middle-third fractures), (*Figs.* 11–14) 28–36
— — — classification, (*Fig.* 11) 30
— — — comminution of orbital floor in, 30
— — — defined, (*Fig.* 7) 17, 19
— — — definitive treatment, (*Figs.* 21–22) 53–58
— — — — fixation procedures for unstable bone, (*Fig.* 22) 54–56
— — — — reduction, 54
— — — — where treatment delayed, 72
— — — incidence, 30
— — — maxillary sinuses involved, 15
— — — orbital floor fractures in association with, treatment, 57–58
— — — signs and symptoms, 30–36
— — — — summarized, 33–34